*Dying Was Not on My Agenda*

by Tracy Stewart

*This book is dedicated to the two most prominent male figures in my life. Dad, I miss you terribly. What else can I say? All those who knew you miss you. You were larger than life, and I learned so much from you—not only from the things you told me, but in the way you lived your life and treated others. More and more people tell me I remind them of you, and even I can see that in myself as my life unfolds before me. I can feel you deeply embedded into the fabric of the man I am today. Thank you for being such a wonderful dad.*

*Dane…buddy…You are the reason I find life so enjoyable. Without a doubt, having you is the best thing I did in this lifetime. I love being your dad and you being my son. You gave me strength when you didn't realize you were. You have been the focus of my journey, and your love carried me to the top of the mountains I have climbed. This book exists because of you. It started as a journal of information to remember me by. It was written to tell you who you are and give you roots to my side of the family. You were so young when we lost Paw-Paw and you've expressed needing to know about the man he was. I hope this book helps to introduce you to him. I also hope this helps you understand my own battles, and why you never knew the significance of it all...until now.*

*"You have cancer."*

With those three words, life changes forever and it changes for everyone you love. I am not certain the human mind can absorb those words—not all at once. Mine couldn't. It is more than devastating; it is more than debilitating; and it is more than heart wrenching.

## STANDING ON THE EDGE

I heard the faint whisper of voices in the room. They were not loud enough for me to make out the words. Some voices were familiar to me, others were not. I was mentally awake, but my eyes were not cooperating. My throat felt parched, raw, and swollen. I could barely swallow. Light slowly creased the slits of my eyes as the room gradually came into view. I felt a clear tube lying across my face that was taped to my nose. As my eyes began to focus, I could see there were other tubes running other places. A pole hung beside my bed with a couple of drip bags pushing fluids into my veins. A machine located somewhere out of view was sounding out *"Beep-Beep, Beep-Beep,"* as it tracked my heart rate. I'd spent enough time in hospitals to at least know that sound. As the anesthesia wore off, pain began to surface. It was a pain unlike anything I had ever known. It was that deep, deep pain felt when a person cuts himself badly with a knife, only much worse. Glancing down at my stomach, my eyes met something hideous; it looked like something from a Frankenstein movie. There were very large staples holding me together. An incision ran from my chest bone to...to forever. The incision was dark blue and the skin seemed to be pinched and contorted by the staples, making the cut look as crooked as a snake ready to strike. For some odd, unexpected reason I thought to myself, *Well, I guess my days of going shirtless are now over.* I blame that on the drugs. It wasn't like those days should not have been over anyway.

I had no awareness of what day it was or how long I had been asleep. Somewhere between anesthesia and pain, there is a state of consciousness that allows a person to know what is happening, yet not be connected emotionally enough to the situation to care. But it didn't take long for it to all start coming back to me...the awareness, the pain, and the emotions. I tried to speak, but I was unaware that the tube connected to my nose actually ran down my throat and into my stomach, preventing me from being able to utter much of anything. My mouth was as dry as a desert, and a nurse was using a teddy bear sponge-on-a-stick to moisten my mouth. I'm not sure why that was so memorable, but it was. The numbness of the anesthesia eventually wore completely off, and the full wrath of pain set in. Once my mind was clear enough to formulate coherent thoughts, I recalled the last thing I could remember, which I presumed to be the previous day. A gastroenterologist, Dr.

Donald Rosen, had told me that I had a very large tumor that must come out immediately. It was discovered during a simple procedure. I had undergone a colonoscopy to investigate what was wrong with me. It was a voluntary procedure, which I decided to have in hopes of preventing cancer. I should have been prepared to hear the news. It wasn't like I didn't know the likelihood that I would eventually have it. Genetically, I was a walking time bomb and I knew it. Despite it all, I wasn't prepared to hear those words, *"You have cancer."*

*"He just needs to get his affairs in order."*—Dr. James West.


## THE CALL

(Four years earlier)

"Dad has cancer and he is in the hospital." Those were the first words my brother, Scott, said to me over the phone that early November afternoon. Just like that—so matter of fact.

"Where?" I know I must have sounded frantic.

"I don't know where it is, I just know he has cancer."

Almost screaming, I replied, "No…No…Where is *he?*"

"RMC Anniston."

It was 1997. Scott and I had not spoken in probably a year, but when we did; we always spoke in those short words that made short conversations. We weren't particularly close, and never had been—not even as little boys. We didn't fight all the time; just when we were close enough to breathe the same air. He was four years older than I was, so I didn't get the best of any of those fights, but I was too proud (or stubborn) to let it go the next time we squared off. That being said, we would fight to the death for each other if need be. So, our conversation was no different that day, but then I don't suppose anything else really needed to be said anyway. I lost track of time for a few moments. I don't recall hanging up the phone or telling my boss that I was leaving work; and I don't remember telling anyone else that I was leaving either. One minute I was walking out of Building 362 at the Anniston Army Depot, and the next minute I found myself driving down the highway toward the Regional Medical Center in Anniston, Alabama. I was trying to make sense out of what Scott had just told me. I could not remember the last time, if ever, that I had seen dad sick.

I just kept thinking, *Cancer…cancer…What does that mean? He has cancer…What kind of cancer? Where is the cancer? How bad could it be?*

I tried to think of others I knew that had cancer and survived. I couldn't think of any. Either there weren't that many, or I was totally oblivious to the fact that some people had actually beaten the disease. I felt ashamed that the latter could have even been a possibility. I didn't let my mind venture far enough to think what I would possibly say to him when I first saw him, or what to expect when I got to the hospital. I just drove.

When I walked into the hospital room, he was sitting on the hospital bed and dressed in a gown. Immediately, I sensed his worry.

"I have a little cancer right here," he said as he pointed to his stomach. His voice was shaky and sad. I wondered what he knew that I didn't. There was no confidence in his voice, and that wasn't like dad at all. I searched his face for reassurance but there was none. We exchanged information about what the doctor had told him and why he had decided to be checked in the first place. I was listening, but so overwhelmed that I didn't comprehend everything that I was hearing. The last time I could recall seeing dad was months before, despite living only twelve miles away. My wife wanted nothing to do with my family, and after each visit a huge argument ensued between us. She finally stopped going altogether, but it didn't prevent an argument between us each time I visited alone. It was an exhausting cycle, and it finally escalated to the point that I rarely visited my family in an effort to avoid the conflict. But on that particular day, I had reason to be upset with him, and I left him standing in his driveway with his head hanging down from a scolding I had given him regarding my own family. I angrily drove away, wedging more of a distance between us than already existed. At that point, it didn't matter at all.

The doctors decided to go ahead and do surgery early the next morning. I reasoned that anytime someone had cancer, it needed to come out as soon as possible. I decided to just stay at the hospital that evening, go home in the middle of the night to take a shower, and then head back to the hospital in the wee hours of the morning for his surgery. I knew that sleep would not find me anyway. As visitation hours ended and late evening arrived, the hospital became quiet—too quiet. Nobody else would be coming to see dad. It would just be the immediate family. The hustle and bustle of people walking down the halls and nurses coming in and out of the room ceased. For some reason, I felt comfort with having people around, even if I didn't know them. Perhaps it reminded me of life in the most downhearted moment I had ever experienced. That night, I sat there in the dimly lit hospital room with so much on my mind that I couldn't seem to formulate one complete thought. It was all I could do to look at dad lying there sleeping—if he was sleeping. I was scared to death for him and wondered what he must be thinking and feeling. I was scared for our entire family too. There was a part of me that wanted that night to last forever. Another part of me was looking forward to seeing the sunrise. It all depended on how this was going to shake out. I wasn't ready for bad news, so I tried to stay positive. That didn't prevent me from sitting there in that room with tear-filled eyes and sobbing as quietly as possible.

Dad's surgery was set to begin early the next morning. I stayed until around 4 a.m., drove twenty minutes to the house for a shower and food, then back to the hospital. When I walked past the waiting area, I could not believe how many people were already there. There were cousins, nieces, nephews, and people from mom and dad's church. The preacher and his wife were there as well. There must have been twenty people in all. I really wanted to be alone or at least with only the immediate family present to gather my thoughts. But those people loved dad, and he loved them. They had a right to be there.

Eventually they told us they had taken him back to start the operation. I felt like I was headed down a hill with no breaks. There was no stopping this ride and getting off. Whatever happened from this point on would be mostly out of our hands. We knew we had several hours before we would know anything, but time slowed to a snail's pace while waiting on word about how he was doing. I don't remember how long it was before they updated us on dad, but eventually they called and said he was doing "wonderfully." I wasn't sure what that meant, but it sure sounded good! I almost felt a big sigh of relief, but something was holding me back. After all, we really didn't know anything. Eventually the surgeon, Dr. James West, came out to a small room that adjoined the waiting room. Mom, Scott, and I were called into the room to listen to what he had to tell us.

Dr. West was an older gentleman—older than I had pictured. His hair was totally gray, and his eyes reflected years of experience in them. He was probably the best surgeon in our area. I searched his face for an answer before he spoke, but I simply couldn't find a clue that would forewarn me as to what he might say. I even remember looking at his hands and thinking, *Those are the hands that we entrusted in saving dad's life.*

Then he spoke to us. "The surgery went fine and he did well. He is a bigger man than I thought he was, but we removed a large tumor in his colon." His voice was calm, confident…almost reassuring. It was a false sense of security that I was feeling. He continued, "He also had several places on his liver that I am sure are cancerous."

"What does that mean, exactly?" I nervously asked the question without knowing if I really was prepared to hear the answer.

His face suddenly changed. His eyes met mine, and then he looked back to mom. The next words he spoke pierced my heart.

"He will need to get his affairs in order." With those words our lives would never be the same.

I felt as though I was going to be sick. My knees wanted to buckle as I reached to steady mom. Her legs lost their ability to support her. I caught her as she was falling, and I eased her into a chair. I turned to find Scott, but he had bolted through the doors, leaving the waiting room and the hospital. I am not sure what he was doing or where he was going. I think he just wanted to run away. Perhaps that was his only way to cope—run. I sort of wanted to run too, but instead stayed behind to face those who had come to see dad. I walked back into the larger room with the twenty or so people that were gathered to deliver the news that dad was going to die. I broke down before I could ever get out the words. Several sobs and deep breaths later, I somehow, some way, managed to speak.

"He said dad needed to get his affairs in order."

It sounded crude. I wasn't capable of considering "tact" at a time like that. Those were the words that came out, and it would have to be good enough. It was the hardest thing that had ever slipped past my lips. I felt helpless, angry, sad, scared, worried, and anxious, all at once. Through teary eyes, I could see the shock on their faces and tears running down several cheeks. Many of those that had gathered walked over to me in hopes of providing comfort and offered their support, but there would be no comforting me in that moment of hopelessness. I was in disbelief, yet hurting at the same time. I was instantly mad at God for allowing this to happen. I wanted answers—and there had better be some good ones.

It took a while for me to gather my senses and eventually realize I had to take care of mom. I needed something to sedate her. Her friend, Willie Cook, was a retired nurse and suggested we head to the Emergency Room. It would be a while before dad would be placed in a room. We walked mom to the ER and got her a sedative. I was acting partly on instinct and partly on a half-cognizant mind. The injection mom received practically knocked her out and certainly delayed a mental breakdown. I was very concerned about how the news would affect mom when the medication wore off. Was she strong enough to go through what was about to unfold in her life? There was reason to worry.

Mom had her problems many years prior to dad's diagnosis. She had severe depression and had to be hospitalized twice. A hard life growing up and losing two babies shortly after birth took their toll on her later in life. The second time she was hospitalized resulted in controversial "shock" treatments. According to her psychiatrist, it was the only alternative for her other than institutionalization. Dad wouldn't agree to have her sent away, so he opted for the treatments and the consequences that came with it. It was an admirable thing to have done. After her treatments, she had been so much better, but I kept wondering, *Can* she possibly handle losing the man she had been with since she was a teenager?

As a way to mask the emotional train wreck I had become, I focused my energy on trying to figure out what to do. I needed to get as much information as possible and as quickly as possible.

*"What are we really dealing with here?"* I kept asking myself that same question over and over.

I started collecting information by calling the patient advocacy contact, which sent an oncology nurse to talk to us. The nurse told me that dad had maybe a year at most "if he responded to chemo." He had less than six months if he didn't.

*Six months…six months…* It just kept echoing over and over in my head.

We had to decide how to tell dad—or even if we would tell dad. How in the world do you tell the man you love and admire most in this world that he is going to die? As a family, we went back and forth as we contemplated telling him, but we ultimately decided to just explain to dad that we were going to approach this as if it were life or death and fight it with the best medicines and doctors we could find. Dad was a smart man and eventually he would figure it out for himself. We all agreed, if he asked, we would tell him the whole truth, but it wasn't a job any of us wanted. It seemed so cowardly to not tell him, but none of us were strong enough to do it. I will wonder the rest of my living days if not telling him was the right thing to do.

Dad would be in the hospital for five or six days. Thanksgiving was a little more than a week away and mom had planned the family tradition of everyone coming to her house for Thanksgiving lunch and dinner. After her mom, Maw-Maw Amos, got too old to do it, she stepped up and started hosting Thanksgiving meals for uncles, aunts, cousins—the whole family. None of us wanted to continue with those plans. Mom wouldn't be up to it, and I am not sure dad would have been either. I was certain dad would not feel like traveling anywhere else if another family member hosted it. Besides, none of us saw much to be thankful for at the time. Our world had fallen apart, and there didn't seem to be any getting it back together. I cursed at God for allowing this to happen to a man like my dad. My prayers were filled with anger, almost condemning God for what He was doing to my dad.

*"He deserved better than this after having served you for so many years! How could You let this happen?"* I got no answer. I honestly didn't expect one either.

Each day I would go to work, then to the hospital until 10 or 11 p.m., and on to the house where I could surf the Internet and search for a miracle that would save dad's life. I became an expert on cancer almost overnight. I read everything I could find to learn all I could about treatments, drugs, experimental procedures, and the best cancer centers in America. No matter what site I went to, I kept seeing the same thing—less than 5 percent survival rate for stage IV colon cancer.

Each time I read it, I kept thinking, *somebody has to be in that five percent—might as well be dad.*

Dad finally went home from the hospital and it was good getting him home. With Thanksgiving dinner at my parent's house canceled and the extended family told to gather without us, we just wanted to spend that time with dad. Mom didn't feel like cooking, but still threw a meal together that would make most families proud. It just wasn't the huge meal we were accustomed to that included turkey and dressing, cranberry slices, deviled eggs, peas, corn on the cob, cream potatoes, baked chicken, sweet potato casserole, cheese cake, and banana pudding. After dinner we all sat in the den struggling for something to talk about that didn't involve cancer. The absence of the extended family was felt like a huge cloud hanging over us, but we realized that having them there would not have changed anything. That day I kept thinking, *this will probably be the last Thanksgiving I will have with dad and he doesn't even know it. I hate that it will be remembered like this.* Try as we did, we just could not make things normal.

We discussed all the options with dad. He seemed to be fine with whatever we thought was best. It was like he didn't want any part of the decision making. It seemed strange at the time, but eventually, it would become perfectly clear as to why it seemed that way. I did my best to inform the family of the cancer research at the major cancer centers, how clinical trials were handled, and where the best doctors were located for dad's kind of cancer. It came down to taking dad to M.D. Anderson, in Houston, Texas. It was the place that seemed to provide the most hope. After calling Houston and talking with the doctors and nurses, it seemed to be the right thing to do. They seemed so confident when they told us to get him out there as soon as possible. The urgency in the voice of the oncology nurse I spoke with seemed to exude confidence. I was so desperately seeking something positive, at least it seemed that way to me.

We made plans to get dad there. Schedules were put into place, time off from work was arranged, and a plan was eventually hatched. We were not sure how long we would be there, or what would happen when we got there. I would be the one to drive mom and dad out there for the first trip. They would have a car if they needed to stay, and I could fly back alone. If they didn't need to stay, I could drive them back to Alabama.

On the morning of our departure for Texas, a small group gathered at the Gateway Restaurant in Piedmont, Alabama. The Gateway was a family-owned restaurant that served as one of the town's favorite meeting places for breakfast or coffee. There were several members of the family and many friends that came to see us off and send well wishes before we set out on our journey. Dad had touched a lot more lives than I had previously realized or given him credit for. It was a testament to his character that people would come out just to see him off. He was a beloved man, no doubt. I was too nervous to eat anything, so I sipped coffee, sat quietly, and pondered what the next several months would hold.

I kissed my three-year-old son on the cheek and said good-bye. I held him as close as I could and whispered, "I love you Dane-Dane. I don't know when I will see you again. I guess I will see you when I see you. I may not be back before Santa comes, but I will be back." I'm sure he didn't understand. I didn't understand it either. It was ten days before Christmas and I might not make it back to watch him open his gifts from Santa. I told the family I would call them as soon as we got there.

As we pulled onto the highway, I felt I would never see Piedmont again. It was as if I was leaving and never coming back. I don't know why I felt that way. Maybe it was just from the uncertainty that life suddenly had presented me with, or maybe deep down I knew that no matter what, life as I had known it prior to that day was never going to be the same again. There was a part of me that felt I was somehow running away and leaving the problems behind. It seemed ridiculous, yet justified.

The drive to Houston took about twelve hours. We hardly talked at all, but when we did, we talked about how our family traveled when Scott and I were little boys. Dad had worked as a civil service worker and drove a calibration van to various military installations to calibrate electronic equipment. Mom followed the van in the family's 1959 Rambler loaded down with about everything we owned. The backseat served as a makeshift bed for my brother and me. It wasn't much fun for two rambunctious kids, but we did get to see a lot of the country. I was too young to remember most of the traveling.

At some point mom recalled a funny story about Scott throwing a tantrum in New York. "Scott was only about four years old when he decided he wasn't going to do any more walking. He sat down on some steps and threw a fit. No matter what I did or said, he wasn't budging. A stranger saw what was happening and decided to come over to help, but he didn't speak a bit of English. He went to jabbering at Scott in some other language, and it scared him to death. Scott jumped up and took off like he'd been shot out of a gun."

I looked in the rearview mirror and noticed a faint smile on mom's face as she stared out the car window. It was the first time I'd seen any glimpse of anything that resembled a smile since the day we received the bad news about dad. We talked about some of the places we visited and the conversation seemed to hinge on those precious years. That era of time seemed to be the most fitting, the simplest, and the most carefree time we had ever known. It was a lifetime ago, but with no complications, no worries, and no cancer. There was a *huge* elephant in the car and nobody wanted to acknowledge it existed. Maybe that was best.

After about twelve hours, we finally arrived in Houston. I don't remember one single mile of that journey other than the limited conversations we shared about those trips we took as a family.

*"What brought you to Houston, Mr. Stewart? Why did you choose to come here?"—Dr. James Wolfe, oncologist at M.D. Anderson.*

## HOUSTON, WE HAVE A PROBLEM

It was 1997 - the same year Timothy McVeigh received the death penalty, a genetically engineered sheep was created named Dolly, and the world lost Princess Diana, Mother Theresa, and Jimmy Stewart. Nothing in the world seemed to be headed in the right direction. It was certainly the case within our family.

A cold December rain fell across Houston as we checked into the hotel. Cars passed along busy streets, one after another—an endless line of headlights that stretched farther than I could see. The rain had little effect on cities the size of Houston. We hadn't been in there more than ten minutes before I realized it was not my kind of town. It was too big and too complicated. I was a small town boy with small town ways. I never wanted to be anything different. My hometown had less than five thousand residences.

More people than that seemed to pass by as I sat at various red lights waiting for them to change. Under different circumstances, I might have been more embracing toward a city like Houston, taking in some sights, going to see a ballgame, or maybe finding some cultural event to attend that wasn't available in Alabama. I had done my share of traveling over the years and was always up for seeing and doing as much as possible when visiting a place I had never been before. Even though downtown Houston was strung with Christmas lights and decorations, I wasn't in a cheerful spirit. In fact, it made me miss home and Dane even more.

We got to our hotel room and dad folded into the bed immediately. The trip had been brutal on his still-recovering body. It was hard on mine and nothing was wrong with me. After being confined in that car for so long, I felt claustrophobic. The walls closed in fast, so I left the hotel to go for a walk. It didn't matter much where the trip took me, and it didn't concern me that it was cold and raining. I didn't even have an umbrella. It was refreshing and helped ease the feelings I was having.

As I left the hotel, I noticed a Salvation Army worker standing near the door holding his bucket and ringing the familiar bell. I reached for some change, but my pockets were as empty as any hope I had for dad. I was not in a generous mood anyway and felt as much in need as anyone who would benefit from the coins jingling inside the bucket. In the back of my mind I thought maybe a good deed would be rewarded with some healing from God. Maybe it was a sign from God—not having any money to drop into that bucket meant there would be no rewards coming dad's way. I wasn't on good speaking terms with God, so any signs from Him would have mostly gone unnoticed anyway. I knew in the past, I'd discovered when I was most in need; it was He that I sought out for answers. I just didn't feel His presence that day.

I plodded through puddle after puddle and temporarily forgot how cold and wet I had become. I lost track of time as I trudged on aimlessly. Finally a peek at my watch revealed I had been wandering the streets for almost two hours. Where had my mindless jaunt taken me? I had no idea how I got where I was or how to get back to where I needed to be. With the realization of being lost, I wondered which direction I needed to head to find our hotel. In my mind I was running; running away from feelings, running away from life, and running away from the troubles that our family was facing. Just like that day in the hospital when Scott ran out, a part of me felt if I could just keep moving; keep running, and not going back, I could outrun them all.

I stopped at a pay phone and pulled out a wrinkled, wet piece of paper from my pocket. The rain had smudged the ink so badly that I could barely read any of the numbers. It was given to me the day we brought dad home from the hospital a month earlier. I dialed the number—partly from memory and partly from the few legible numbers left on the paper. I had looked at the piece of paper a thousand times over those few weeks, wondering if Houston was the place where we would find hope—if not a miracle.

"Hello?"

The voice on the other end of the line was not familiar to me. It wasn't the Alabama dialect I expected to hear. It seemed more refined and proper. I suppose that is what happens when you leave the town you were raised in.

"Judy?"

"This is Judy…"

Judy was a friend from high school who had made her way to Houston years earlier. We graduated from high school together, and I had not talked to her or seen her in many, many years. She had called my family when she heard about dad and gave us her telephone number in case we needed anything while in Houston. Though we had lost touch over the years, possibly life and death had reconnected us. She had come to Houston for the same reason I was there. She moved there when her mother was diagnosed with terminal cancer. But, Judy never came back to Alabama. Death and sickness created a life for her there, and she stayed. I was hoping "life" would be the reason I would return to Alabama. We talked for a while—mostly about how we ended up in Houston, and we did a little catching up on each other's lives. I can't say I felt much better about dad's situation after we talked. Still, it was nice reconnecting with someone I had once known and who had made the same journey I was on. Maybe I was looking for some sense of "home" or maybe I just needed to talk to someone that had walked the same path I was walking and had made it through, good or bad.

I looked around for anything that looked familiar and started finding my way back to the hotel. By the time I returned, night had settled in and it was getting late. I hurried up to the hotel room and slipped the keycard into the door, dreading what was on the other side. I knew the room contained an ominous presence. My escape was about to come to an end—no more running. It was time to face it all and get on with it. As I opened the door, the lights from the adjoining bathroom were casting a dim light across the room. In the shadows, I saw my father sound asleep. He was tired. I think it was more from the emotional battle of dealing with cancer than being physically tired from everything that had happened. Mom had snuggled as close to him as she could get, trying to cling to him as much as possible. I wasn't sure if that was a normal thing for them to do. I had a feeling it wasn't. I hadn't seen the two of them sleeping in bed since I was a kid across the hall. The circumstances had created a new bond with them that I wasn't familiar with. They never showed a lot of public displays of affection—not even at home, but that was changing. I didn't know who needed it more, mom or dad.

I began to think about how they had been together almost fifty years—since they were teenagers. Dad was only fourteen years old when they first fell in love. She was almost a year older. They ran off and got married when they were sixteen. It is unique these days for marriage to last that long, especially one that started at such an early age and began with eloping. They had to love each other very much, or they were too ignorant to recognize they didn't—or too stubborn to call it quits.

Back in the day, dad could have easily been one of the characters known as a "Greaser" from the movie *The Outsiders* with his slicked back hair, rolled up jeans, and plain white t-shirts.

His dad was the local town mechanic and had a reputation of being a booze drinking, womanizing, mean-spirited man. I'm not sure if it was rightly deserved or not. I was only eighteen when he died of Hodgkin's disease, so I never really got to know him. I do know he didn't provide much of a home life for dad and his brothers.

Dad's mom, a God-fearing, hard-working, Christian woman, did the best she could to instill a sense of worth and family values into Dad and his three brothers.

The boys would work on cars in their dad's garage as a means to have their own transportation and a little spending money. The boys were known for driving fast, racing, and were even rumored to have done some bootlegging from time to time on the back roads between Piedmont and Georgia. If they sound like the typical Southern outlaws that were the genesis of NASCAR, they probably were.

Dad wasn't the kind of boy mom's parents would have chosen for her—far from it. If America had subscribed to arranged marriages, dad would have been in the back of the line. Mom's dad pretty much hated my father in the early years, offering to shoot him if he came to pick mom up for a date. That didn't stop them from seeing each other. It probably didn't help any that dad would sit outside their house in his car and peel rubber on a regular basis, sending plumes of smoke into the air like a drag racer at the starting line. But over the many years of their marriage, the feelings mom's parents had toward dad would change. He would be loved like a son before all was said and done. Once people got to know dad, he just sort of had a way of winning them over. They were no different. He would become the first person mom's parents reached out to when something needed to be done like work on a vehicle, or fix something in the house that had broken or needed replacing.

But times were tough in those days, and the only chance of getting out of that little town of Piedmont was by joining the military. Each of dad's older brothers had joined, so he was certainly expected to do the same. The only thing that may have prevented him from joining was Gerald—the brother closest in age to dad—who was killed in Korea. He stepped on a land mine in a place named "Old Baldy." When they brought him home, only half of him was left. Dad, at age fourteen, went with his dad to identify the body. But dad still joined the Air Force a few years later.

Certainly mom and dad's marriage was far from a perfect one. They had experienced more than their share of heart wrenching events early on. While dad was stationed for basic training in Biloxi, Mississippi, mom lost her first baby, Rodney Thomas. There were complications at birth, and he died after living only a few hours. Mom was still living in Piedmont, so dad returned home to bury their child. I am sure it was a tortuous drive. After the funeral, Dad took mom with him back to Mississippi, then on to Victoria, Texas, when he was re-stationed.

It must have been so difficult on both—especially being apart when Rodney died. I am sure they needed the strength of each other at a time like that. But life's misfortune wasn't through with them. A year later mom became pregnant with their second child, Kermit Wayne. Like their first baby, he died shortly after birth due to complications. This time, mom was confined to the hospital after delivering the baby. Mom and dad both wanted the babies buried next to each other in Piedmont, so dad drove all the way back to Alabama with Kermit's body inside a tiny casket in the back seat of his car. Dad had to bury him alone—with mom being hundreds of miles away. I simply can't imagine the pain he must have felt and how challenging that must have been. And, I can't imagine mom all alone while her baby was being buried without her. It amazes me how they stuck together through so much tragedy.

And now, many years later, in their golden years, they were facing yet another heartbreaking moment in their lives. Mom and dad needed to believe there was a chance—at least a slim one. I felt it was my responsibility to give them one.

Looking at Dad as he slept, I noticed he looked older than I had ever seen him. I never thought of him as being feeble. He was short in stature but a strong, stocky, man. He was athletic—even into his forties and fifties. The man I was seeing now seemed to struggle with every step and pant with each breath.

As soon as I could shed the wet clothes, I climbed into the shower and made the water as hot as I could stand it. I just stood there, trying to think of nothing and wanting more than anything to escape the thoughts that consumed me. The water ran down my face in a continuous flow. I couldn't wash the feelings away that encompassed me, and I couldn't soothe the chills that were bone deep. I finally made my way back into the room, and I pulled the desk chair next to the window. I stared into the traffic and city lights below. I was miserable and antsy as I peered into the darkness. Gaining my focus, I noticed my reflection in the glass. It cast a portrait of tears rolling down my cheeks, which flowed in unison with raindrops on the glass. I couldn't tell which ones were raindrops and which ones were my own tears, but they all felt like the latter.

I started recalling every memory of dad I could conjure. Maybe I was trying to hold on to memories of him before they got away, or maybe I just thought of the possibility of having a limited number of memories left to make with him. I decided to start at the beginning and think back to the earliest moments I could remember and move forward through my life. There were so many memories I had mentally shelved over time—mostly from my childhood. They were becoming more precious as I reflected upon them. A floodgate opened and I could remember intricate details of things from my childhood. It was amazing how vividly those memories came to me. I thought about camping trips with the Adderhold, Martin, Johnson, and Ledbetter families over at Little River Canyon and Coleman Lake. Even specific trips and events unfolded as if they had just happened the day before. More than anything else, I thought about the years dad spent coaching youth baseball to so many kids in Piedmont. It was probably how most kids would remember my dad, and where he made the biggest impact in the lives of others. We practically lived at the ballparks growing up. I had more than my share of dinners filled with hotdogs, pickles, and snow cones, but they never got old. Looking out that hotel room window, I could almost smell the cotton mill as it burned off cotton, and see those enormous oak trees that surrounded the fields. It was a simple time and those days were golden. In this moment, nothing seemed truer than when Robert Frost wrote "Nothing gold can stay."

*God apparently has a plan for us, and many times He uses our entire lives to prepare us for the battles ahead.*

## SWING AWAY

It was obvious dad was in for the fight of his life. Lying there in bed was a man that was immortal to me, like a superhero that nothing could harm. He was incredibly smart too. I thought if anybody could beat this cancer, it would be dad. He was such a competitor and hated losing. Maybe sports and coaching should have been his real calling.

Dad coached many of the youth baseball teams Scott and I played on. Even when he wasn't coaching the team, by the time the season rolled around, dad would somehow work his way into the dugout and onto the coaching staff. He would manage to get a matching hat and shirt. Before the season ended, the other coaches would be following his lead as if he were the head coach. Dad was a very good coach—a smart coach, but more than anything, he made it fun. Maybe that is why both kids and adults loved him so much. He could teach kids, and they weren't even aware they were learning. He knew how to do little things to teach kids how to hit, catch, and throw, yet never losing sight that it should be fun. Dad would sometimes lay bats on the ground around a batter to teach kids not to step outside the box when the pitch was thrown. If a kid stepped out, his feet would roll on the bats making him fall. It was unorthodox, but effective. As kids, we would laugh at each other, but it accomplished what dad had intended. Even at home, he would work with Scott and me on little things that made huge differences. I remember him taking me to the city park in Piedmont for batting practice. We marked tennis balls with colored markers. He would have me call out the color on each one as he threw it. He was a natural at coaching and knew how to teach kids what to do. I wondered how a man whose dad shared none of those things with him as a child could have been so good at working with kids. Kids loved playing for him, but I know he loved coaching them more.

Growing up in a small Southern town, there wasn't much else to do except enjoy local sporting events. It was free to watch and since most of the people that lived in Piedmont were "mill villagers" with limited incomes, anything free was a godsend. Those ball fields provided an opportunity for people to socialize with someone other than their neighbors and served as a nucleus for the community.

Dad would load up kids into the bed of that '69 Ford pickup and haul them all over Piedmont, trying to get them to and from practice and games. He knew some of those kids couldn't have played had he not been the taxi for them. He didn't mind driving miles out of his way to give a kid a ride home. Many times kids that lived only a couple of blocks away would ask for a ride home. They saw him as a father figure and just plain loved the man. His generosity didn't end there either. Dad always seemed to have shoes or an old glove for some kid without them.

As those sweet memories continued to surface, I thought about one of my first at bats as a minor leaguer. I must have been about seven years old, standing at the plate with the bat resting on my shoulder. Some kid was hurling a ball that seemed to be traveling one hundred miles per hour, and he didn't seem very consistent in where he threw it. In those days, there were no batting tees or coach-pitch leagues, so getting hit by a pitch was near certainty. There were seven-, eight-, and nine-year-olds tossing the ball to the plate, so anything close was a strike. But, there I stood in that batter's box with that bat in my hand, resting on my shoulder. I wasn't thinking about hitting the ball at all. I was thinking about that ball hitting me. This wasn't dad throwing tennis balls, this was some kid I didn't know throwing something much harder, and I was scared to death. The kid had thrown a few pitches—two of which were called strikes, but not because I swung at either.

"Time Out!" dad shouted from the third-base coaching box. I walked over and he put his hands on my shoulders and said, "I don't care where this next pitch is thrown, I want you to swing at it."

"What if it isn't a strike?" As if it mattered. I hadn't swung the bat yet.

"Just swing at the next pitch." He was calm and assuring as he spoke.

I was certain somehow that dad knew the next pitch was going to be a strike. If I swung at it, I was going to hit it. I didn't question him at all, so I swung at it—and I missed it. To this day, I don't know where that pitch was thrown, if it was a ball or strike, or how close I came *to* hitting it or how far I was *from* hitting it. What I do know is a seven-year-old finds little value in striking out. I was embarrassed and angry. How could dad have been so sure that I should swing? How could he do that to me? It never occurred to me that I may have struck out had I *not* swung at the ball. Nor did it occur to me that even had the pitch been a ball, I still may have hit it by swinging. It took thirty-one years for the epiphany to occur. Dad wasn't teaching me about baseball at all; he was teaching me about life. He was teaching me that it is sometimes better to swing and miss than not swing at all. He was teaching me that if I go down—go down swinging. That lesson molded future decisions and was an instigator of my actions so many times in life. It would become the most important lesson for me to remember a few years down the road.

But as fun as dad made sports, there was also that competitive side that he demanded from us boys. He could be too competitive sometimes—at least I thought so. He wanted us to put everything we had into something, no matter what that was. Early on, that competitive attitude was new to me, especially when I first started playing ball. I vividly recalled one minor league game while I was playing for the Red Sox. We were playing the Tigers that Saturday, and my best friend Carlton was playing third base for them. Dad was coaching third base, and I had somehow gotten on base and made my way to third. I was no more into that game than any of the little kids in the stands were. As I stood there talking to Carlton, I didn't notice the crack of the bat when the ball was hit. I didn't hear dad yelling for me to run either, so I didn't run and I didn't score. The next player struck out, and my actions cost my team one run. Dad grabbed me by the arm so hard he lifted my feet off the ground as he dragged me to the dugout. He was not happy that I had cost my team a run. I was not happy with him. I was told to park my rear end on the bench the rest of the game. But looking back, there was a lesson to learn from even that. Maybe he was saying that if I am going to participate, then go *all* in and go *all* out. Maybe it was a lesson in humility, or one to show that other people would sometimes be counting on me to do my job. Only in my thirties could I see the value in that. It wasn't the fondest of memories, but still a cherished one as I sat there sifting through the moments that had shaped me.

The teams that dad coached or helped coach won about seven or eight league championships. When the seasons were over, dad often loaded the teams up and took them to see the Atlanta Braves play. We would ride all the way to Atlanta and back, packed in a truck or a car like sardines, and it was the most wonderful experience imaginable. It may have very well been the highlight of some of those kids' lives. I didn't realize it then, but I would be willing to bet my paycheck that dad picked up the tab for anyone that couldn't pay—if not for all.

Even in the later years of our youth-playing days, with many years of his coaching ingrained in us, dad would still find ways to contribute. A smile came across my face, sitting there in that Houston hotel room as I recalled the day dad showed up for practice one afternoon, while I was playing as a fifteen-year-old in the Babe Ruth league. That team was very talented, and the season would end that year with a perfect 20-0 record. Half of those games ended due to the "Ten-Run Mercy Rule." The team had two excellent pitchers, John Coley and Jeff Formby, and both were nursing sore arms. The head coach needed someone to throw to the batters and dad gladly volunteered. Years earlier he had been a fast-pitch softball pitcher and somehow never lost the ability to throw. Scott and I knew it from playing pitch and catch with him, but the other kids were amazed. His pitches were every bit as fast as any we had seen, and they were being delivered in a totally different way. We swung and swung at his pitches—batter after batter. As good as we were, we were no match for his pitches. As each player took his turn, the other players would laugh at how foolish each batter looked trying to hit "the old man's pitches." One player, a super-talented athlete named Moon River Ridley, was certain he could hit off him. He strutted to the plate as if he were about to show us all up. Like the rest of us, he fanned air that day as well.

Even though dad could no longer coach me when I reached high school, he would still come to the games and walk to the fence if he ever saw me on deck.

"He throws high…watch the curve on the first pitch…make him throw you a strike first. He hasn't thrown a strike on the first pitch all day." Dad always had some advice and he was rarely wrong.

Over the years, dad lived his life mixing a rare blend of fun and competitiveness. He always wanted to come out on top—to be victorious and have fun doing it. It didn't matter if he was playing tennis, golf, or Rook, he wanted to win. He loved to compete. It was deeply rooted within him, but I'm not sure from whom or from what. In spite of the fun-loving prankster he was, he would lay the nonsense aside and get down to the business of competing when game time came. Now, he was facing one of those times— only this wasn't a game, and losing meant everything.

I was in this with him…all in…100 percent. His qualities had been ingrained into the very fabric of the man I had become. We could not afford to lose this one. It simply wasn't an option. Cancer was in for a fight till the very end. If God had a plan, I was hoping He would reveal it to me or at least help me prepare for what was to come.

At some point in the wee hours of the morning, I made my way to the bed and drifted off to sleep.

*I had become an expert on colon cancer. I knew more about the disease than most general practitioners. I knew all I ever wanted to know about it, and then some.*

## THE TREATMENTS BEGIN

The next morning, we walked over to M.D. Anderson. As we entered the lobby, I wasn't sure we were in the right place. Nothing about that place looked like a hospital. The front door opened into a multi-floor foyer made of nothing but glass. The sunlight illuminated the place and served as the official greeter for the patients and employees. Off to the left, a lady was playing a baby grand piano. The tunes resonated throughout the entire area like a concert hall. People were scurrying about everywhere. We sat there in amazement. I was thinking, *This is M.D. Anderson? Are we in the right place?*

As we sat there taking this all in, we noticed bus after bus pulling up and letting people off. Each bus that pulled up was full. It didn't take long to figure out that these people were coming for treatments. The bald heads and masks gave them away, but otherwise, these people really didn't look sick. That vision provided some hope, but I was overwhelmed that so many people had cancer, and this was just one of many comprehensive cancer centers. There were eleven others across the country. I had no idea that many people had cancer. It was obvious that cancer didn't discriminate either. There were people of all ages, color, nationalities, and sex.

Dad said, "I am sitting here noticing that ninety percent of the people here with cancer are younger than I am. I guess I have been looking at this all wrong. I should be wondering why I was able to live this long and *not* have cancer." It was a unique observation—one that I am not sure I would have made in his position.

M.D. Anderson is certainly a wonderful place. It is said you only get one chance to make a first impression, and we were impressed. We were certain this was the right place, but we also knew we had not seen a doctor, and no doctor had seen dad. We twisted our way from station to station as we processed in—finally

making it to where we needed to be. We met with an oncologist,

Dr. Robert Wolfe. He was a very calm and confident man. We

talked with him about treatments and what could be expected from

the drugs that dad would be taking. Not once did he seem hopeless.

He spoke with an assuredness in which I found comfort. I realized

I knew much of the language he was speaking. From the research I

had done, I knew the road he was putting dad on. I asked a few

questions that obviously indicated I wasn't some dumb hick from

Alabama that didn't know how to read.

"Once we get these tumors in his liver shrunk down to five

centimeters or less, I would like for you to call the University of

California at San Francisco. They are doing an experimental

treatment called radiofrequency ablation."

Doctor Wolfe looked at me and grinned. "I see you have

been doing research. I certainly will do that. I have a colleague that

is participating in that FDA Trial and will be glad to refer your dad

to him."

Dad looked over at me somewhat surprised. I think he realized for the first time that I was totally in this with him—all the way. I didn't tell dad everything I had researched and discovered—only what I thought he would benefit from. I wasn't about to give up or let him give up either. Still, I felt a little guilty sitting there thinking, *I know what the chances are of him surviving five years with stage IV colon cancer. It is less than five percent. I know Dr. Wolfe knows that too. But dad doesn't know.* Part of me was scared Dr. Wolfe would spill the beans. Part of me would have welcomed it finally coming out, but thankfully it never did. The remainder of the day was filled with tests and blood work, and on the following day were CT Scans. We finally finished up late that second afternoon.

We would not know anything for a couple of days, so we took the opportunity to have one day to try to forget about why we were in Houston. We decided to visit the zoo since it wasn't too far away. The weather was fairly nice that day, so it seemed like a great way to spend the day. Arriving at the zoo, the closest parking spot I could find was about 200 feet away from the entrance. We parked and started walking. I immediately recognized dad's pace was considerably slower than mine—and slower than his normal pace. He was struggling, and I could tell his breathing was labored. We made it just inside the gate, and dad looked as if he was close to collapsing.

Through his panting he said, "I need to sit down."

I gathered he was feebler than I ever imagined. I realized he wasn't immortal after all. Cancer had become his Kryptonite. We never really saw the zoo. We packed it up and returned to the hotel and dad slept most of the day.

The following morning we made our way back to M.D. Anderson to meet with Dr. Wolfe. He informed us they had decided on a drug called 5-FU. It was a drug that had been around for forty years and there really hadn't been any new drugs developed that were any better. Dr. Wolfe knew the distance from Alabama to Houston might prevent dad being treated there. M.D. Anderson agreed to call the shots from Houston, letting dad get his treatments back home in Anniston. He would only return to Houston for CT Scans and examinations. We called the family back in Alabama and notified them of the plan. When we left Houston, dad seemed to feel better for having taken the journey, but for me—not so much.

As soon as we got back to Alabama, I hit the Internet. I don't know what I thought I could possibly find that I hadn't already discovered, but I could not quit looking.

I had researched 5-FU and I knew it might work for a while, but eventually it would stop working. If there were no other drugs that were any better, then what would we do? I kept thinking, *We can put a man on the moon but we can't come up with a cancer drug any better or newer than 5-FU?* I decided to learn everything I could about the National Institutes of Health and clinical trials. It is the last ditch effort, the end of the road, the place to go when there are no other places to look. I knew it would come to that sooner or later. The NIH is a federal government entity responsible for overseeing all new trials for drugs and procedures. We were just buying precious time with the 5-FU and M.D. Anderson. At the same time, it was scary to think that the federal government could soon be calling the shots, knowing how they operate. I worked for them, and while I depended on their paycheck, I would not want to depend on them for healthcare. I searched the ongoing clinical trials. Some seemed barbaric, trying to test the toxicity doses on humans, while others seemed to be a crapshoot with very poor odds. Many studies would be blind, using a placebo for some of the patients. I could not believe there were people, thousands of people most likely, going up there for treatment and not getting any of the drugs they were testing. How hopeless does one have to be to take a chance on possibly getting a drug that might work or to allow some procedure to be performed on them that may kill them in the process? There were so many people in desperate need of a miracle that there was never a shortage of patients willing to try anything. Each of the studies I read about had qualifying and disqualifying criteria: "must not have had 5-FU drug or CPT-11" or "must have failed all conventional treatments" or "must not have CEA levels over 5." It was a sea of information that had to be whittled down until a small list of possible treatments appeared that dad might actually qualify for. The more I read, the more I hated cancer. I wasn't exactly happy with God at that moment either.

Soon, I discovered chat rooms and discussion groups on the Internet where cancer survivors and caregivers were sharing a wealth of information. There were actual people that I could chat with who knew what worked and what didn't! I was so excited I had found another source of information and hope! I signed up for many of the discussion groups and read the posts more and more often. Unknown to me, there was a society of people that existed who was pounding the chat rooms and forums doing exactly what I was doing—looking for a miracle. How could these people exist without me even knowing about them? I felt ashamed that I was so naive or uncaring to have not known. The people and cancers were so numerous that the groups and rooms had to be broken down into smaller groupings by cancer types like colon cancer, pancreatic cancer, or brain cancer. I had never thought about how cancers are actually different and that the drugs and treatments would also be different. I was wrong in believing that "cancer is cancer." There are an endless number of possible outcomes from patient to patient. Finding something specifically for dad was like looking for a needle in a haystack—a haystack that was being continuously added to. The people in those discussion groups seemed about as knowledgeable as some of the doctors I had met. Most were cancer survivors, and many currently had active cancers. A few members were loved ones searching for answers just like me. "Knowledge is power," so they say, and having the Internet can be a wonderful thing—or a terrible thing. I kept noticing that some of the people in the chat rooms who had been posting for weeks and weeks would suddenly stop posting. Their posts might be informing the group of some experimental treatment or clinical trial and then weeks would pass with no posts. It was concerning. These people became friends, brought together by a common foe and sharing the same plight. Occasionally, someone on the forum would comment that the reason the posts had stopped was due to the poster succumbing to their disease. It was heartbreaking and it happened over and over again.

I kept asking myself, "Why do I put myself through this?"

Looking into dad's hollow eyes made me realize I didn't have a choice. Each day I would get up at 5 a.m. to prepare for work, work all day, get off work, and drive fifteen miles past my house to Piedmont. There, I would spend a couple of hours with dad, then I would head back home around 9 p.m. and surf the Internet until the wee hours of the morning. The next day, I would do it all over again. I was exhausted, but quitting wasn't something I could live with.

Eventually, I began calling doctors and nurses that were contacts for several clinical trials. I spoke with medical personnel at the University of California at San Francisco, Dana-Farber, Sloan-Kettering, the University of Alabama at Birmingham, and Duke University. I contacted the National Institutes of Health and discovered there was a new drug that was about to be approved called CPT-11, which would eventually be known as Camptosar.

Over the next year, dad did pretty well on the 5-FU. He would have some of the more common side effects like weakness and peeling of the skin on his hands and feet, but otherwise he was able to get out for light activities like church or dining. During that time, we tried to get dad to eat healthy and to keep him well hydrated, which is critical while taking chemotherapy. There were several trips back and forth to Houston for CT scans during that year for evaluations. Mom, Scott, and I took turns going out with dad.

By November of 1998, it was my turn to accompany dad back to Houston. I had seen dad slowly deteriorating over that year and knew it was a matter of time before the chemo would stop working. It had been a year, and the words from the oncology nurse that dad had maybe a year if he responded to treatments echoed in my mind. I worried about what they would tell him. We met Dr. Wolfe in the hallway as we were being escorted into an examination room by his assistant.

"Ya'll come over to the slides; I want to show you something."

We walked over to a large wall full of panels where scans were being read. He pointed to dad's slide and said, "Mr. Stewart, this is your liver and these spots you see are the tumors. This other slide is what your liver looked like when you came to see us the first time. As you can see, there were seven tumors, and now there are only three."

I was too cautious to allow any joy to seep in. I had a feeling there was a "but" coming somewhere in Dr. Wolfe's explanation.

He continued, "We have been able to shrink the other four tumors, but these three have stopped shrinking."

And there it was, the "but."

"How big are these tumors?" I asked. I was thinking about the possibility of dad getting radiofrequency ablation treatments and Dr. Wolfe knew it.

The confidence and assurance was no longer present in his face as he looked me square in the eyes. "Eleven, nine, and seven centimeters. Those are too large for radiofrequency ablation treatments."

Dad had been quietly standing there while we talked medical terms and then he asked a question I wished he had never asked. "What does this mean doc?"

I felt a lump in my throat because I knew the answer. It was a moment I will never forget. Somehow Dr. Wolfe must have sensed that dad didn't realize the terminal condition he was in, and that I probably did. We made brief eye contact as if to say, "How am I supposed to answer that?"

He turned back to dad. "Mr. Stewart, we have thrown the best drug we have available at your cancer. There are other drugs that are less effective, and harsher on the body. It is up to you if you would like to try those, or if you want me to get you into a clinical trial, I will. But, I have to tell you that eventually the cancer will catch up to you."

Dad turned to face me and his eyes met mine. I am sure mine were filled with tears. I wasn't sure what his look meant, but I felt I had betrayed him in the worst way. I had become Judas. He must have been thinking, "Tell me you have an answer since Dr. Wolfe doesn't. Please tell me you can help me." I was helpless and speechless.

We left M.D. Anderson that day, knowing we would never return. It was a somber trip back to Alabama, and I had no idea what to say to dad during those hours on the trip home. If our conversations struggled before, they were practically nonexistent for the flight home. We came back to Alabama feeling defeated.

The week after we returned, dad opted to try the other drug Dr. Wolfe mentioned. M.D. Anderson switched his infusions to Camptosar and called the shots on doses and frequency from Houston. An Anniston oncologist, Dr. Ellen Spremulli, would administer the drugs. When the first treatment of Camptosar was given to dad, he landed in the hospital two days later. He had constant diarrhea and could not eat. He was sick for days. In his already weakened state, it almost killed him.

When we finally got him home, dad told us, "I don't know how much time I have left, but if the quality of life I have left is up to taking that drug, I don't want it anymore." We were running out of options and running out of hope.

I had been reading about some other options, even home remedies that might help dad. I ordered him some shark cartilage because there was a crazy ad in some cancer newsletter that read, "Sharks Don't Get Cancer." It was their selling point. Dad wasn't a shark, but we tried it anyway. The fishy smell made dad sick, which prevented him from drinking it. We were desperate enough to try anything, but every avenue was a dead end. Every second we weren't fighting, the cancer was winning. I knew the end would come quickly if the cancer wasn't being treated. I just didn't know exactly how quickly. His body had already been through so much, and I wasn't sure what he could endure in such a weakened state. I continued to pound the Internet, sleeping only two or three hours each night. His fight had been going on for over a year and this was my lot in his battle. I was meant to do this, despite the toll it was taking on me mentally, emotionally, and physically. I had once believed everything happened for a reason. I was no longer sure that was true.

*"Okay dad. I will take care of mother—but right now, how about you let me worry about taking care of you?"*

## THE FIRST PROMISE

Dad had taken his last chemo in early December of 1998. Shortly after the Christmas holidays, during the wee hours of the morning, I got another momentous phone call. This time it was from my sister-in-law, Becky. She informed me that mom's brother, Jerry, had suffered a massive aneurism and wasn't expected to live. He was in the hospital in Atlanta, Georgia, and mom and dad had headed to the hospital ninety miles away. It was the last place dad needed to be, and the last thing he needed to do.

I told Becky, "I'm going to get dad and I will bring him back."

I threw on some clothes and a baseball cap and headed for Atlanta to retrieve dad. The minute I walked into the hospital waiting room I spotted dad. He was slumped over in a chair, barely able to hold up his head and resting it on mom's shoulder. He looked pitiful. Jerry was like a brother to dad, and I understood why he wanted to be there. Dad was so weak and sick that it didn't take much coaxing to get him to leave with me. A man my dad loved like a brother was just down the hall and was expected to die, but dad was ready and willing to leave. He knew he had bitten off more than he could chew. I said my well-wishes to the family, hugged my aunt and mom, and headed home with dad. Mom stayed behind, so it was only me and dad for the two-hour trip home. On the way, I struggled to find things to talk about. It was much like the last Houston trip, but we were much further into his cancer journey now. I was reluctant to say anything to dad about more treatments. The feeling kept nagging at me that I was pushing dad through painful treatments due to my own selfishness. I knew the final outcome would be the same regardless. I just wanted to keep him around as long as possible. I finally announced to dad that I had found a doctor in New York that was doing some experimental treatments, and I had already spoken with him.

I explained, "He thinks he can help you dad. It's a pretty serious procedure, and it isn't FDA approved yet, but he would like to take a look at you. I'll send copies of your medical charts to him and we can go from there. I also called mom's aunt and uncle in Long Island and they said you all can stay with them while you are there!"

In his weakened voice he replied, "I am not going to New York, Tracy." And that was that. He was done. He was tired of needle pricks, tired of worrying, tired of feeling badly, and tired of being tired.

He shifted his conversation to cars, finally expressing how he wanted to trade the old Lincoln Town Car in for something small and economical—maybe a foreign car that was more reliable.

Unaware of where this conversation was going, I asked, "Dad, do you really think this is the best time to worry about trading cars?"

With a heavy look, he replied, "Your mom needs a car that is dependable, and she has a hard time with that big Lincoln."

It hit me that dad was trying to do what Dr. West told us he should do over a year earlier—he was getting his affairs in order. A lump came to my throat the size of Texas, but I just kept driving—unable to speak.

He continued, "I want you to promise me that you will take care of your mother. I need you to make sure she is okay and do things for her that I would do. She is going to need someone to do those things."

I finally managed to mutter, "Okay, dad. I promise I will take care of mother—but right now, how about you let me worry about taking care of you?"

That was all that was mentioned about the promise I made to dad, but it indicated to me he knew he was dying. Suddenly there was a bond I sensed with him that had never existed before. I don't know why, but I had never felt like dad's favorite. We'd never had the ideal father-son relationship, and I wasn't sure he was proud of me for anything I had ever accomplished. He never said so, so maybe that was it. He was not a man of endearing words. It wasn't how he was raised, so it was not natural for him. I suppose he did the best he could, considering his own experiences growing up. But now, sitting in the seat next to me was a man that had never uttered the words "I love you" to me, nor had I said those words to him—at least I could not remember them ever being said between us. I knew dad realized that I had known all along he was going to die. He knew I kept fighting for him, researching, calling, pushing, and trying to find a miracle where there was none. He knew I was someone he could lean on and who would do what I said I would do. He knew I would take his place and fulfill the promise to take care of mom after he was gone.

When we got home and I got him settled for the night, I helped him into the house, then into bed. I was tucking him in, just as I did my five-year-old son.

As I turned out the light, the words parted my lips without effort. "I love you dad."

He told me he loved me too. It didn't seem odd or contrived. It seemed senseless that we had never had that exchange before. Maybe it didn't seem to be the manly thing to do, but that didn't matter to me anymore, and I was certain it didn't matter to him either. It was something that we never failed to say to each other after that day. I went back downstairs and looked around at all the photos and collectibles they had sitting around. There was a lifetime of memories in that home, and honestly, it made me realize there were some things missing in my own life.

A few weeks later, dad tried another round of Camptosar as palliative treatment for pains within his liver. The results were the same—maybe worse. By February, he finally relented. He didn't want to die—he was just tired of living life as it was.

By April of 1999, I had started building a house and was having the basement poured when my family called from Piedmont. They told me if I wanted to see my dad before he passed away, I needed to come right away. It was a call I had known was coming since the day we talked with his surgeon seventeen months earlier, yet I was not prepared to hear those words. I had become so task oriented and mission driven to search for a cure, I had not allowed much time for grieving. I had not stopped long enough to ponder life without dad or how his death would change my life. Maybe that was my way of coping, or maybe I knew somebody had to pick up that ball and run with it—or maybe both. It was April 17—a date that meant nothing before…a date that would mean everything to me from that day forward.

I made it to Piedmont that morning, and I decided that I would not leave his side until it was over. It had been several days since dad had really been responsive to anything or anyone around him. The weeks preceding those days, dad hallucinated and talked to people that weren't there but ignored the people that were there. His liver was shutting down and the ammonia level in his body caused hallucinations. I could smell the ammonia oozing from his skin. He was suffering so much, and I could not imagine what he was going through. I was so angry at God for allowing anyone to suffer such a horrible death—especially my dad. Where was He?

Where was the God I was brought up to believe would be there in our greatest time of need? Where was the miracle worker that could heal men and bring the dead back to life? I simply didn't feel like turning to Him for strength after allowing this to happen to someone I loved so much. I didn't feel like He had been much help to dad up to that point and didn't figure that was going to change anytime soon. I wasn't deserving of an answered prayer, and I knew it. But dad was.

Late in the evening dad's breathing became extremely shallow. His eyes had been focused on the wall, looking straight ahead, not blinking, and not changing his focus to anything else. He had been like that all day. He seemed to be waiting on something or someone. Up to that point, I had never accepted letting him go, but his suffering had endured much longer than it should have. I made my way to the head of his bed and bent over him. I placed my arms over his shoulders, like I was hugging him from behind. I pulled his head to my lips and whispered in his ear.

"Dad, remember when we were coming back from Atlanta you asked me to take care of mom. I promised you I would. Remember? Do you remember dad? I will dad. I promise. It is okay to let go. I will make sure she is okay. Just let go."

I worked my way to the side of his bed and held his hand. Less than ten minutes had passed when he made one last gasp, his eyes turned down to the right, and he had the most pleasant look on his face. He was seeing something we weren't. He was almost smiling. Maybe he got his first glimpse of Heaven, or maybe Rodney and Kermit—the sons he never got to know. I am not sure what he saw, but I am sure he saw something. And with that, I said, "I love you dad" one last time. I reached up to shut his eyes. I like to think dad heard those words. Dad lost his battle and succumbed to cancer just before midnight. He did what he had always taught us to do; he went down swinging.

The moments following dad's death are hard to explain. At first, there was some sense of relief that dad was no longer suffering. I felt numb and defeated. I walked outside and sat in the middle of the road, folded my arms over my knees, and laid my forehead on my crossed arms. There was a house full of people, and most seemed to have "someone" to comfort them. Yet, there I was alone. It spoke volumes to me concerning my own marriage. Eventually, dad's older brother Chuck must have realized I wasn't in the house and made his way outside to find me.

He reached down and placed his hand on my shoulder, "You all right?"

I gave an affirmative nod, but the grief that others had been burdened with day to day, a little at a time, suddenly came crashing down upon me all at once. It was overwhelming.

Looking back, his death seemed so senseless. He was a smart man and I just kept thinking. "Why didn't he get a colonoscopy when he was in his fifties? *That* is what they tell men to do! How could he not have been smart enough to know that? He was such a smart man!"

The next day was filled with funeral plans, picking out a casket, and selecting pallbearers. I was going through the motions, making decisions with my brother, but I couldn't tell you what those were. The funeral director told us we had to pick out something to bury dad in. When I got to mom's house, I went upstairs to her and dad's bedroom. I opened his closet doors and just lost it. For the first time, I let it all go and just sat down in the floor and cried like a baby. I was picking out the last thing my dad would ever wear. Somehow, I muddled through it and found a nice navy suit. Mom always said she loved him in navy.

Dad was laid to rest on April 20, 1999, in Highland Cemetery in Piedmont, Alabama.

*"I am pretty sure what you have is Giardia. I am going to give you a prescription for an antibiotic, but we'll do a colonoscopy anyway."*—Dr. Donald Rosen, July 2001.

## THE DIAGNOSIS

After dad passed away, I made a conscious decision to change my life-style, stop drinking alcohol, eat healthy, exercise more, and lose some weight. I was thirty-six and too young to be worried about cancer, but I wasn't willing to take any chances. I went to see my family practitioner, Dr. Michael Herndon. I explained that I wanted to be checked for colon cancer. I knew it was often hereditary and explained that my dad and uncle had both been diagnosed with colon cancer. He didn't hesitate to refer me to a specialist.

It seemed stupid to be so young and asking for a colonoscopy. It was sort of like asking someone to drive splinters under my fingernails. The stakes were high, so I wasn't about to gamble with my life or repeat the same mistake dad made. For him, he could claim he didn't know better, but for me, it would just be pure stupidity. I knew at some point I would need to address possibly having the disease.

I was referred to a gastroenterologist, Dr. Pankaj Kashyap. I didn't expect much from the visit. As I explained why I wanted to be checked, he pressed around on my stomach, asked a few questions, and then quickly informed me that I didn't need to be checked until I was forty. He went on to explain that my father wasn't diagnosed until he was in his sixties, and my uncle was in his seventies, so he didn't see a need to go through an invasive procedure at such an early age. Only 4 percent of colon cancers are discovered in patients under forty. I felt I would be safe for a few years, and then maybe get serious about further testing when I turned forty.

The next year passed quickly as I buried myself into my job and getting ahead in life. I had put my life on hold for seventeen months while helping dad, and I had some catching up to do. I was putting in some serious hours at work and neglected my health and everything that was wrong in my personal life despite my decision to be healthier. The time I wasn't spending on my job, I was spending it with Dane. I was very active in the community serving as a PTO officer and a member of the Parent Advisory Council at his school. I also served on the Youth Athletics Board during this time.

One afternoon I stumbled upon a photo of me receiving an award at work and noticed I had gotten fat. I am not sure how or when it happened or why the mirror had been so untruthful to me over the years, but I was fat all the same.

I still had a clean bill of health from the year before, so it was time to make some healthy changes. I purchased a cheap mountain bike and started taking five to ten mile rides on the Chief Ladiga Trail. The Chief Ladiga Trail is a "Rails to Trails" project that converted unused railroad tracks to a paved walking and riding trail. It serves as a hub for joggers and cyclists and provides a perfect environment for each. It was nothing strenuous, since the maximum incline is only four degrees. I wasn't blazing any paths on my short rides, but it was a start. I also changed my eating habits by removing red meat and all fried foods from my diet. Soon I began losing weight and dropped from 188 pounds to about 170 in just a few weeks. Even though I was getting in shape, I was feeling tired all the time. I looked healthy but didn't feel healthy. I didn't want to admit that something was possibly wrong with me. I credited it to being thirty-seven. How does a person know how a thirty-seven year old is supposed to feel if they have never been that age before?

The first inkling that I was really sick was in October of 2000 while attending a Halloween party. I wasn't feeling my best, but I went anyway. During the party, I began feeling sick and was sure I was coming down with strep throat. I was freezing from fever and chills and left early. When I got home, I climbed into bed hoping my fever would break. My fever was almost 103 degrees, but I didn't make a big deal out of it with my family. The next morning I felt like I had not gotten sick at all and passed it off as some twenty-four hour bug.

Two months later, I was sent to Washington, D.C. to attend a two-week training course on technology. The trip was the most miserable trip I have ever experienced. It was bitter cold, and I wasn't feeling well from the moment I exited the plane. During the second week in D.C., I had another bout with a high fever, accompanied by diarrhea. I was convinced I had been food poisoned from eating sushi with three colleagues. The diarrhea was off and on for the remainder of the trip. Each afternoon, I went straight to the hotel, climbed into bed, and went to sleep.

When I got back to Alabama, the diarrhea continued for several months. I had turned thirty-eight during that time. Even though my dad had similar symptoms when he got sick, I didn't even contemplate my situation being anything more serious than a bug. I reasoned that since I had seen a doctor to be checked for cancer, I was fine. It had to be something else. Soon, everything I ate made me sick, and I was spending most of my time going to the bathroom. I made another appointment with my family practitioner, Dr. Herndon. He remembered sending me to a gastroenterologist the year before and now he was aware of my family history of colon cancer. He ordered a FOBT, or fecal occult blood test, to check for blood in my stool. I took it home, completed the tests, and took it back to his office. He told me he would call me if there were anything to report from the tests. Before the test came back, I spotted blood, and I knew I was in trouble—big trouble. It wasn't bright red, indicating that the bleeding was farther up inside my intestinal track. It was a sure sign of colon cancer and I was scared to death. Could cancer have found me too? Surely I didn't have it! I called Dr. Herndon back and told him what I had discovered. Immediately, he sent me to a different gastroenterologist, Dr. Donald Rosen in Jacksonville, Alabama. I had an appointment within a week. The day I met with Dr. Rosen, he assured me he thought I was fine and was almost certain what I had was *Giardia lamblia,* a bacteria that invades the intestines and causes similar symptoms. He gave me a prescription for antibiotics then sent me on my way. As I was leaving, he added, "I still think we need to schedule a colonoscopy—just to make sure."

I went back to see him the next week for a follow-up and to schedule the colonoscopy. The antibiotics had done the trick. I wasn't sick at all and was feeling better than I had in months. I was considering cancelling the colonoscopy, but Dr. Rosen still thought it was a good idea and gave me the instructions for the procedure.

The colonoscopy was scheduled for 7 a.m. two days later. I spent the next day trying to keep down that Phospho soda, which I could only describe as being like an entire canister of Morton salt mixed with castor oil. What didn't go straight through me almost came back up.

When I arrived at the hospital for the colonoscopy, Dr. Rosen reassured me as I was about to fade off to sleep. "I am sure you are fine. It was probably just a bacterial infection."

There I was having the most dreaded procedure imaginable. I was scared of the procedure and scared at what the outcome might be. I was equally scared of not having the procedure. I knew if this turned out to be cancer, waking up on the other side of this procedure would be the beginning of hell for me. They rolled me into a room and asked if I wanted to be "put all the way to sleep" or just "sort of out of it." One look at the contraption that was about to enter my body in places where nothing should be, and it was an easy choice. I wanted to be *out* for this one! I would be awake within an hour or so, and I could get on with my life—or so I had hoped.

Anesthesia can be a godsend. Not necessarily because of the numbing effect it provides for the body, but the numbing effect it has on the mind and emotions. As it wore off, it allowed me to slowly become cognizant of the world around me, providing "teaspoons" of misery as the numbness subsided. It was then I heard those words, those dreaded words, the same words my dad heard a couple of years before.

"Mr. Stewart, you are one lucky man to have gotten checked. You have a stage III tumor in your colon and it has to come out *now!*"

I simply didn't understand what Dr. Rosen was telling me. Lucky? Tumor? Who, me?

*Merriam-Webster* defines cancer as *"a malignant tumor of potentially unlimited growth that expands locally by invasion and systemically by metastasis"* which doesn't even begin to sum up what it really is. A more appropriate way to define it would be "a potentially deadly disease that consumes the body, mind, and spirit, and releases demons from Purgatory on anyone who has it."

I won't lie; I was scared to death. Not of death, but of a fight that I knew I had little chance of winning and what it would do to those who had to sit by and watch me lose it. My family was zero for four with this disease. The thought of dying at thirty-eight consumed me immediately. Well, not so much the thought of dying, but of not living. I know it sounds the same, but it really isn't. Standing on the ledge between this life and the next isn't something a man can comprehend until he is teetering between the two. At that moment, I wasn't thinking of the process of dying or what would actually happen five seconds before or five seconds after I died. I wasn't thinking about any reconciliations I needed to make with God (and I had some coming), or standing at the Pearly Gates waiting to get in, nor was I thinking about how painful my last breath might be or the loss of dignity that comes with the last stages of the disease. Instead, I was thinking about things I would never get to experience again, and the things I would never get to experience even once. I had fleeting thoughts about rainbows and skies filled with rain, about sleeping late, going on vacations, watching sunsets, fishing, and laughing. But mostly I thought about missing time spent with those that I love—especially my seven-year old son, Dane. *Oh, God, Dane!* It became all I could think of. I didn't realize how much I loved life until that moment, but I knew how much I loved him. I wanted to do nothing more than to savor the good things in life and the things I love about life. As I reflected and made mental lists, the reoccurring themes racing through my mind were, *"But I may not get to do that again"* or *"I won't ever get to experience that."* There were so many thoughts, I could never focus on just one. All were gloomy. There was so much life to live and so many things I hadn't done yet. I wondered, *Is it downhill from here? Is this the best I will ever feel again, until my last dying breath?* I envisioned Dane growing up without me, and the moments in his life I would never get to share with him or have the opportunity to see him do. I wouldn't get to coach him in youth sports the way my dad coached me, never get to take him to school, or watch him grow up. I knew he wasn't old enough to have many lifelong memories of me. At seven years of age, most memories would fade before he had kids of his own. His kids would never know me. While my mind raced out of control, my heart was broken into a million pieces. I was an emotional basket case inside, but I knew I didn't need to appear to be. I needed to be strong, but I feared I wasn't brave enough to face the days that may be coming, nor strong enough to face dying. This was real. This was happening. I had never been so close to dying and yet felt more alive. I never thought the two could go hand in hand, but they do.

Only days before, I was muddling through life focusing on my career, vehicle payments, mortgages, bills, and taking care of my family. I was living an average life, but I still had a lot of living to do. Dying was not on my agenda. Suddenly, nothing else mattered but being alive. It wouldn't take long for me to realize that facing death would test my courage, my faith, and my will to survive. I realized that I wasn't appreciative enough of the life that had been given to me. And, here I was at that place, with one leg over the fence. Everything that was important to me before suddenly didn't matter, and things that should have been important to me all along were all I could think about. My world had been turned upside down.

I was recovering from the colonoscopy in the Jacksonville Hospital and I knew the drill that followed. It was all too familiar to me. I knew a five to six day stay in the hospital would be required to allow my body time to heal. I knew all about this cancer that was growing inside of me, and I even knew the medical term for it—adenocarcinoma. I knew exactly how the cancer progressed in one's body, the survivability and prognosis of each stage, the drugs used to treat it, the radiation treatments that are often required, and what those treatments and drugs would do to my body. Worst of all, I knew how it could eat at the body until there was nothing left to eat. I had studied adenocarcinoma in the colon for years. I knew that the only drug on the market to treat it was the same drug that had been used for the previous thirty-plus years. Despite colon cancer being ranked third in cancer-related deaths, science had not found anything new that was better than 5-FU. It had only been two short years since my life had been consumed with trying to find a cure for my dad. The only thing I didn't know about cancer was what it was like to have it myself and be forced to fight it with every ounce of my will. I also didn't know that the fight I was about to undertake would isolate me from the world and leave me feeling like other's lives were continuing without me.

Dr. Rosen went on to inform me he had a surgeon already lined up. His name was Dr. Dwayne Clark and he was supposedly hand-picked by none other than Dr. James West—the same surgeon that operated on dad. It seemed like history repeating itself. I had been diagnosed with the same disease that had taken so much from me.

I thought to myself, *"When is enough, enough God? What do you want from me?"*

I didn't go into this diagnosis as blindly as dad did. There wasn't anyone having to decide if they would tell me or not, or what the potential outcomes might be. I knew exactly what I was facing.

Before the anesthesia had worn off, I was being rushed around the hospital for preoperative tests. They performed blood work, gave me a barium enema, and administered a CT scan before the day ended. I had already been prepped for surgery with the colonoscopy, so the surgery was scheduled for the next day. They were pushing to get this cancer out before it did any more damage to my colon walls.

Dr. Clark came by to tell me he would be doing a colectomy. He explained to me that my cancer was pretty low in the colon and there would be a good chance I would have to wear an ostomy bag for the rest of my life after the surgery. It was enough to make me want to cry.

Early the next morning the nurses came to get me for the surgery. They placed warm blankets over me as they wheeled me toward the operating room. I was unconscious within seconds and never remember entering the room.

In what seemed like minutes, I awoke in the mentally delusional state of anesthesia and began my personal journey with the disease that had taken my grandfather, father, uncle, and first cousin—the latter three within the previous two years. I wasn't prepared for any of it, but I knew there were two options—fight or fold.

The next few days were hell and emotionally draining. All I did was worry about Dane. He was only seven years old. He was only five when his paw-paw died two years earlier, but he knew it was from cancer. I couldn't tell him that cancer was what was wrong with me too. It was too much for a kid that age to handle. I didn't want to take away any of his joy of being a kid by worrying about me. So, I made the decision to not tell him. It was heart-wrenching thinking about not being around to see him grow up.

It was a Thursday, and it would be a few days before the pathology report would be available. Dr. Clark thought it would be Monday before he would know if he got clean margins with the surgery or if there were any lymph nodes involved. I knew from my research that if there were some lymph nodes with cancer in them, I was stage III, and if not, stage II. The survival statistics would be decreased from 50–60 percent to about 30 percent.

For the next several days, I went through the grueling task of getting up several times a day and walking as far as my legs would allow. I was determined that I was not going down without a fight—just like dad. I had a seven year old at home depending on me to be there to raise him. And then there was that "other" seven-year-old kid…back at the plate and dad was telling me to swing away. I had little hope for a different outcome. Dad was a better man than I would ever be, and if he couldn't beat it…well…you know.

The hardest part of that weekend was waiting on that report to come back; the easiest part was hitting that morphine pump and going back to sleep as often as it was programmed to work. It was the only peace I could find. Even with as much pain as I was experiencing, I was hitting the morphine pump more to prevent dealing with the emotional side of having cancer. When I was awake, the same questions ran through my mind. *Were there any lymph nodes involved? Were the margins clean at the incision marks? Were there any signs of metastases?* It was basically going to be a life or death verdict not unlike a prisoner waiting on a decision for the death penalty.

Monday night rolled around and I was feeling somewhat better—physically anyway. I was still depressed and worried. That night a nurse came by to inform me that Dr. Clark was in the hospital seeing patients and was coming to see me. Like a dog waiting for his master to return, I kept watching that hospital room door wondering when he would appear. I was thinking how I was going to try to read his face when he walked in. If it was bad news, how was I going to respond? The suspense was terrible. I was expecting a death sentence and having to decide how to handle it. It seemed like hours before he came walking into the room. As soon as Dr. Clark walked in, he was smiling from ear to ear. I barely remembered what he looked like after only meeting him once before the surgery. He looked so young, too young, but that smile on his face made him look even more so. He reminded me of a kid that had just done something incredible. I was hoping he had.

Dr. Clark burst out, "I can't hold it in any longer. I have to tell you that your margins were clean and none of the lymph nodes we took had any signs of cancer in them. Congratulations!" He went on to inform me that I would not have to wear a colostomy bag for the rest of my life, which was fabulous news.

It was like a weight had been lifted off of me. Not that I was out of the woods, I just wasn't in the woods as deeply as I could have been. I knew that my chances of beating this were drastically better with that news, but were still about the same as a coin being flipped and landing on either heads or tails. Fifty-fifty odds are great in Las Vegas. Life, however, is different. But I would take it!

Dr. Clark made me an appointment for a few weeks later with oncologist, Dr. Helen Spremulli. She was a cancer survivor herself and the oncologist that administered dad's chemo for M.D. Anderson. The parallels between my life and dad's life were uncanny.

At first, I was thinking that I might not have to have any chemo at all. Dr. Clark even indicated it was a possibility. For me, a couple of weeks seemed too long to wait for a doctor's appointment. So I also made another appointment at the University of Alabama at Birmingham (UAB)—thinking I could possibly get to see an oncologist sooner. However, it would be after my appointment with Dr. Spremulli before UAB could see me. Nobody seemed to be in a hurry to help me get on with this cancer fight, and I was thinking how every minute counted. I selected

UAB for the second opinion because it was a cancer research hospital, much like M.D. Anderson. It was close to home, and their reputation was among the best in the country.

The day of my appointment with Dr. Spremulli, I was wondering if she would remember dad. I wasn't particularly pleased with her bedside manner with dad, but she had such a great reputation as a doctor, that I really didn't care. When she walked in, I will never forget her words to me: "Well, it looks like trouble for you."

*Trouble? Trouble? What did that mean?* I wanted to hear how she was going to treat me and beat this cancer. I needed encouragement.

She spoke so matter of fact. "I am going to treat you with six weeks of 5-FU. My assistant will make you an appointment with a radiation oncologist, and also schedule your infusions." A few strokes of the pen and she walked out.

I remember thinking, *That's it? That is my oncologist? Trouble?* I simply could not seem to get the idea that I was just a number and just another patient, out of my head. I wanted it to matter that I was a person or at least have the perception that it did. Maybe it was just a very bad day for her, but I was committed to see what UAB had to say anyway.

I opted to hold off on starting chemo until another doctor could see me. A couple of weeks later, I made my way to UAB. I was assigned to an oncologist in the hematology department of Kirkland Clinic, Dr. Robert Posey III. I met with Dr. Posey and immediately knew that UAB was where I needed to be. He was a young, African-American doctor, and was very personable and intelligent. He had a great bedside manner, and we hit it off like two peas in a pod. He talked to me about other things. He wanted to know all about what I liked to do and what I thought about things. I had learned with dad's treatments that it is always better to be a "person" and not a statistic when you are talking to doctors. Surely a doctor would be more diligent in trying to cure me if he cared about me as a person.

I told Dr. Posey, "Look, I don't care what you throw at me; I want to be as aggressive as possible with this. I don't care what I have to do. I have to beat this. Not beating this isn't an option." He must have taken me at my word. He recommended I have a subcutaneous port surgically placed in my chest and have it connected to a 5-FU chemo pump for six weeks while I received twenty-eight radiation treatments. He wanted to follow that up with another fourteen weeks of continuous infusion of 5-FU with the pump. It was so much more than what the other doctor had recommended. Twenty weeks seemed like forever to be connected to a chemo pump, but I signed up without a second thought.

The next week I had a port surgically inserted into my chest, which included a round, disk-shaped object inserted below the skin that would receive the needle. A tube was connected to it that ran up into my jugular vein, then on to my heart. I left the surgeon's table and headed directly to Dane's football practice. I was determined that cancer wasn't taking more from me—not if I had anything to say about it. Looking in the mirror that night, I stood staring at this ugly lump residing behind yet another scar. My body looked like I had been in a war. In a way, it had been.

Later that week, I was given instructions to visit an outpatient clinic to have my chemo pump connected. I walked into the clinic and met Cheryl, a nurse with an excellent attitude and such a sweet disposition. I felt comfortable with her being my assigned nurse. I removed my shirt, and she pulled out a kit that included a needle shaped like an L. It was as large as pencil lead, and was painful when it was inserted into my chest. Connected to the needle was a tube that ran into the chemo pump. She explained how the brick-sized pump would provide chemo to my body around the clock, and I would have to return each week for a refill, needle change, and to have my dressings changed.

Most, she said, wore a fanny pack and placed the pump in it. I laughed and stated affirmatively, "Me with a fanny pack? I don't think so! Even if I have to tote the stupid thing in my hand everywhere I go, it would beat a fanny back!"

No offense to men who wear fanny packs, but if I wasn't already feeling like less of a man, a fanny pack would be the nail in the coffin. Enough was enough!

She handed me a spill kit—complete with rubber gloves, suit, mask, goggles, and a hazardous waste disposal container.

Shocked, I asked, "This is what you are pumping into my veins? Something that comes with a Hazmat kit for hazardous spills?"

She laughed and said, "Yes, but this is *good* stuff."

I bantered back, "I'm sure that depends on the perspective of being the pumper or the pumpee."

I thought to myself, *Well, it has started. This day will be the best 'feeling good' day I will have for a* long, long, *time—if I ever have another one at all.* I never realized how debilitating a thought like that could be, but overcoming the emotional obstacles are part of beating cancer…maybe the hardest part.

I purchased an elastic rib protector, which had Velcro straps to hold it in place. I simply placed the pump just under my armpit on my side, where it would reside for every waking hour except when taking a bath. I wanted to hide it as best I could. Cancer was already going to take away most of my dignity. I resisted it whenever I possibly could.

*"We're going to put plus sign tattoos on your buttocks to serve as markers for the alignment of your external beam radiation treatments."—UAB radiation technologist.*

## IT BEGINS

Youth football had begun, and Dane was among those participating. Going out in public was different than it had been before my diagnosis. Some people were overly friendly that had never been before. Were they genuinely concerned, or were they thinking they didn't want the bad karma to bite them in the rear end for not being nice to a dying man? Other people that were considered friends before my diagnosis, suddenly acted like they hardly knew me. Was it because they didn't know what to say, so they avoided me altogether, or did they just write me off before I was ready to kick the bucket? Maybe they were afraid they would catch it. I'm sure for most, there were no motives behind any of it—it just made me wonder. Having cancer made me feel like a leper—unclean and diseased. I was sure people sitting around had heard about my cancer. I could see their heads turn my way and hear their whispers as I approached people gathered in groups. Maybe they weren't talking about me. I don't even know why it mattered, but it did. I wasn't sure what they had heard, or what they knew to be factual. I didn't need sympathy; I needed normalcy. I wanted someone in this fight with me like I had been with my dad, and I wanted more than anything to wake up from this nightmare.

On the Friday of the week my port was installed, I went for my radiation "markup." I had no idea what that was, but they explained the need to tattoo my hips, buttocks, and lower back with plus signs that would be alignment points for the external beam radiation. So, now I was going to have tattoos on my body. Great, just great! If I was going to be getting a tattoo, I wanted something cool, not some mathematical sign that probably looked like it was done in prison.

At the markup session, I was asked to strip down and was instructed to lie face down on a narrow table. A large machine that had red laser beams emitting from a long pivoting arm rotated around and over my body. A female technician drew "plus signs" with Sharpies over my hips, buttocks, and lower back. Thank goodness they weren't permanent tattoos! The technician drew the signs where the red-beamed crosshair reflected on my body. The machine hovered above me and moved back and forth like a large robot arm. The technician kept shifting me until I was perfectly aligned on the table. It had to be the same for each and every day radiation would occur.

The treatments began the day of the markup. I wasn't expecting it, but was ready to get this over with. For each treatment I would be nude, lying face down with my rear end shining like a harvest moon. The technician would have to shift me left, right, up, and down until I was perfectly aligned with the laser beams, which meant I was going to be mooning this female technician for fifteen minutes at a time for the next twenty-eight days. Of course, humility goes out the window when someone has cancer, but it doesn't get any more humiliating than being nude with large scars running across your body and an ugly port that looked like a large acne bump under the skin on your chest with tubes connecting to it. It was not a pretty sight.

After my first scan, I met Dr. John Fiveash, my radiation oncologist. Now I had *two* oncologists. Dr. Fiveash was wonderful also. He had a good bedside manner and was very down to earth, much like Dr. Posey. I also made a personal connection with him, as I learned that he had triplets that were seeing an occupational therapist at the Bell Center at the hospital. It just so happened, I had a friend from high school that worked as an occupational therapist there and worked with his kids! I would make sure I would always ask about them. I had to keep those personal connections going. Dr. Fiveash explained what would be happening to me, what to expect from the treatments, and what he expected the outcome to be. It sounded like they were going to be burning my insides up, and that was exactly what the plan was.

The weekend was one of anxiety and sadness. I felt less than human. Monday came way too soon, but I began the remainder of my twenty-eight treatments. I was shocked that I didn't feel anything while the treatments were happening or even afterward for that matter. Radiation occurred from Monday through Friday, so I knew this was a six week ride I was on.

Each weekday that followed, I reported to the Lurleen Wallace Tumor Center, named after former Governor George Wallace's wife. Since it was a very strict regimen, the same people were there each day. Each time, I would undergo my five to ten minute alignment, followed by five to six minutes of radiation. In the waiting room, I became friends with many people, striking up conversations about our cancers and our lives. It's weird, but names didn't seem important at the time—only that we were kindred spirits fighting the same enemy. I wish I had written down their names now and kept in contact with them. Four of the most prominent people that I met included an older couple from Opp, Alabama, and a mom and daughter from Talladega, Alabama. The older man had pancreatic cancer. He seemed healthy when I first met him, but he passed away before his treatments were over. The young girl from Talladega was undergoing radiation for pain management or palliative treatment.

Her rather young-looking mother told me one morning, "She doesn't have long. She is a senior in high school, but she isn't going to make it to graduation, and she really wanted to graduate."

My heart sank. All that kid wanted was to graduate from high school, and here I was still pissed at God for losing my dad and feeling sorry for myself. My direction and attitude changed that day—at least in my approach to my treatments. I was still angry with God. I was there to possibly be cured, and even though I might be there to get palliative treatments *one day,* it wasn't *this day.*

The next couple of weeks passed without much indication anything was going on except being a little more tired than normal. I was even working six hours a day. But by the fifth week, things became drastically different. I no longer had the strength to walk from the parking lot to the waiting room without a rest. I wasn't even able to walk normally and shuffled my feet like a feeble old man. It felt as if my entire insides would fall out if I took one long stride. If you ever watched Tim Conway play the old man on the Carol Burnett show—that was me. I was going down and going down fast. I could no longer work, nor could I stay out of bed for more than a couple of hours at a time. I was pretty much confined to the house. There is an element of cancer that is very isolating to people who are battling it. Going out in crowds with a debilitated immune system is not advisable and friends often worry their phone calls are bothersome. Having a very close personal relationship with someone or a spouse who can share the burden of cancer is essential. Since Dane was too young, it only left one person to fill that role. But we never had conversations about my cancer, or me dying, or what life would be afterward without me. A counselor told me in the beginning that cancer could make a relationship stronger or it could create a distance in the relationship. One thing for certain – it would never be the same. It didn't take long to figure out which would be the case for my situation. Some people simply aren't strong enough to deal with someone close to them having cancer. Those that have cancer aren't given a choice.

The treatments continued and my health continued to wane. Many days Dane would asked me to get in the floor and play with his action figures, but after a few minutes of play time, I would become too exhausted to continue. At times I would lie down on the sofa and reach down to the floor to play with him. He was the center of my world and cancer had taken away my enjoyment of playing with him. I wasn't about to steal his childhood with the knowledge I was fighting for my life. His contribution in supporting me in my battle came from his constant requests for me to play with him. It kept me going more times than he knew.

Eventually, the treatments became so severe I would go home and go straight to bed afterward. I wasn't sure I was going to be able to make it all the way through the treatments before they killed me and the cancer wouldn't have to.

The last weekend of radiation, my brother-in-law was getting married in Gatlinburg, Tennessee. I had to decide if I was going to try to make that trip or not. Since the entire family was going, and I had become estranged from my own family, there wasn't going to be anybody to take care of me if I stayed behind. I was afraid that something might happen and there was no way I would have been able to drive myself to Birmingham. It seemed like the smart thing to do was to make the trip. It was a terrible decision and a regretful one. The five hour trip was way more than I could stand. Just being alert for the ride exhausted me. When we got to Gatlinburg, I crawled into bed and didn't leave it the entire time we were there. To make matters worse, five weeks into my treatments, I had begun experiencing short-lived but very severe pain in my tailbone that would come and go. The doctors couldn't imagine why it was happening and had no explanation for it. It was excruciating and so bad that I would jump to my feet and grimace as if someone was torturing me with fire. To cope, I would get to my feet and walk the pain away. On the trip, we had to stop the car on the side of the interstate, and I would walk around until the pain subsided.

The week after the trip, I was back at UAB getting my last three treatments, which were different than the previous twenty-five treatments. Those last treatments were called a "boost," which were even stronger radiation treatments than before, but confined to a specific area. Thankfully, those would come with fewer side effects. As soon as those were over, I was disconnected from the chemo to give my body a rest. The port, unfortunately, stayed in for the next round of chemo. It wasn't long before I started feeling half-human once again. But, that would only last about four weeks, as the chemo pump was reattached. This time there would be no stopping for fourteen weeks.

A week after returning from Gatlinburg, I was scheduled for CT scans to see how things were going. The CT scans would all be the same, with accompanying lab work early in the morning, followed by drinking three large cups of a liquid that tasted like metal to prep for the scans. The CT scans with contrast dye would follow, then an appointment with Dr. Posey. After that appointment, I had a post-radiation appointment with Dr. Fiveash. It was an all-day event.

At my first post-radiation appointment with Dr. Posey, he came in to talk to me and excused himself for a few moments, leaving my medical chart behind. I opened it and began to read. *Extreme swelling in the area of resection. Thickened areas are possible indications of recurrence.* The radiologist was indicating they suspected a recurrence already? When Dr. Posey came back and read the chart, he didn't mention the specific language about recurrence. He only referenced the need to watch the area closely where my colon was reattached.

Later that afternoon, the words written by the radiologist were weighing heavily on my mind. I had to know exactly what his concern was and how certain he may have been regarding a recurrence. My appointment with Dr. Fiveash would give me a perfect opportunity to ask the question. It was almost a relief when he told me, "Of course there is swelling. I'm burning you up inside, and the layers of your colon are getting burned off little by little. Don't worry about a recurrence. There is only a twenty percent chance that a recurrence would occur locally." What he didn't say was that the other 80 percent of recurrences were distant recurrences, and much more difficult to treat. Most of the time, it would be the liver where it metastasized.

The weeks came and went, and the chemo began taking a cumulative effect on my body. My hands and feet would peel and burn constantly. I lost my fingerprints because of the excessive peeling on my hands! I felt as though I had lost something that I knew made me, me. Cancer was even stealing my identity. By week twelve, I began having a severe burning sensation in my neck. It was like a lit match being held to my skin. Dr. Posey assumed my chemo was leaking out, which was very dangerous, so he ordered a sonogram to find the leak. They didn't find a leak, but they did discover that pushing that wand on my neck resulted in me jumping straight up off the table in pain. Next, they ordered an ink injection and X-ray. Oh boy! More radiation! They found nothing. Finally, one of the nurses happened to notice that one of the sternocleidomastoid muscles appeared to be pulling or protruding outward. This, they reasoned, was a result of scar tissue in my chest pushing my port away from the sternocleidomastoid muscle, which is what anchored the tube before it ran into my jugular vein and to my heart. They wanted to surgically remove the port with only two weeks left in my chemo treatments. As badly as I wanted that port removed, I decided that I had ridden it out for twelve weeks, and there was no way on God's green earth I wasn't going to keep it two more. Advil and I became good friends for a couple of weeks and I pushed through it. The same week I finished my chemo, I had my port removed.

It was late February 2002, and I was done! All that was left were CT scans from here on out and a life to get on with!

*"If God had other plans, the only promise I would have broken would have been to myself."*

## THE PROMISE OF AUSTIN

I had spent my time recuperating from surgery and overcoming the chemo and radiation by reading Lance Armstrong's *It's Not About the Bike*. The book was a gift while I was in the hospital, and a welcome escape from worrying about cancer. It was good therapy to realize a person could come back from cancer and become the greatest cyclist the world had ever known. I wasn't a cyclist, but it gave me an idea. I made a promise to myself that if I could ever get past the effects of the radiation and chemo treatments and be healthy enough to ever ride a bike again, I was going to get a road bike and start cycling. My destination would be Austin, Texas, to ride with Lance in the annual Ride for the Roses weekend. Lance had created the ride as a benefit to raise money for cancer survivors. I started researching the ride and discovered there were twenty-five, forty, seventy, and one hundred mile events. I decided on the one hundred mile ride. It seemed like a pipe dream anyway—might as well do it right. I even started telling people about my plan, knowing it would paint me in a corner. I would have to go or look like I was either lying or making something up. I know people thought the cancer had gone to my brain, or that I was on some serious medication when I told them I was going to participate in a one hundred mile bike ride…in Austin…with Lance. I was a weakly, dried-up cancer patient that did good to get out of bed and walk through the house. I still had chemo and radiation hurdles to overcome, and I was planning this trip as if nothing was wrong with me. The truth was, I needed something to occupy my mind from thoughts of dying. I needed to promise myself that I would go, promise myself that I would be healthy enough to ride it, and promise myself that I would be at a given place at a given time in the future. If God had other plans, the only promises I would have to break would be to me. I didn't figure it would matter much at that point.

I got my hands on a nice road bike in April of 2002, loaded it up in my truck, and headed to the Chief Ladiga Trail for my first ride. I wasn't sure how it was going to go. It went much worse than I expected. I could barely crank the pedals—even in the easiest gear. There were people jogging faster than I was riding. It was even more embarrassing that I was laboring for every breath as I poked along. I made it about three miles and I was spent. I had lost down to 154 pounds and was still reeling from the effects of cancer treatments. I didn't expect to be so weak.

The Chief Ladiga Trail became a daily visit for me, and I eventually started riding on the roads of the Pleasant Valley Community near Jacksonville, Alabama. I knew I had to get accustomed to climbing hills before I headed out to Austin, Texas to ride in the hill country. But riding on the rural roads of Alabama presents some unique challenges. Few motorists are aware that Alabama law gives cyclist the same right of way as a car. The roads' shoulders are usually too narrow to ensure a cyclist's safety. Since Lycra cycling shorts aren't exactly accepted attire in rural

North Alabama, most people that saw me on the roads didn't know what to think of me in my cycling gear. I'm certain I was the brunt of many jokes, but I couldn't exactly train under the radar. People in the community knew it was me. There were no other cyclists riding the roads where I trained daily. Good ole boys driving by in pickup trucks would regularly see how close they could come without actually hitting me. On one occasion, I had a beer bottle thrown within a couple of inches of my head and a truck mirror strike my elbow on another. As dangerous as it was, I was determined to accomplish what I said I was going to.

Cycling brought a focus and peace to me that I can't explain. The Lance Armstrong Foundation (LAF) ride had been rescheduled from spring to October to prevent interference with Lance's training for the Tour de France. There was no way I was going to be ready by October that year. I was starting in too big of a hole. It would take me months to get back to square one. It would be the following October before I could get to where I needed to be. At least it gave me more time to train. I just didn't know if I had that much time left to live. Still, I rode as much as possible. Work at the United States Attorney's Office had changed significantly since I had been hired two years earlier. Federal agencies became aggressive toward prosecuting public corruption and white collar crimes. The amount of paper created from those type cases demanded electronic discovery and altered how we prepared and tried cases. Electronic discovery fell under the umbrella that I was responsible for overseeing. The demands at work were overwhelming, but a welcomed distraction from having cancer. By the time I arrived home from work, I was in need of some serious physical activity and would head out on the bike as soon as possible. There were summer days that were so hot and humid that they left me depleted and dehydrated. When I would return from these rides, I would sprawl out in the living room floor and not move for hours. Even on stormy Alabama days, I would ride during the rain and thunderstorms. I figured God had his chance to take me already. Lightning and thunder would not be his *modus operandi*. The winter days were so cold my hands could barely hold on to the handlebars and left me aching to the bone. Over time, I learned to love the elements. They made me feel more alive.

Riding came with a cost, however. With every pedal stroke came guilt of not spending time with Dane. Riding gave me a sense of fighting back against my disease and having some control over it. It became a reflection of life in ways I would have never imagined. Coasting down hills was like the times when life flows effortlessly and everything seems to be going right. Long winding hills began to represent life's struggles. They were often too large to envision overcoming them without focusing on one pedal crank at a time.

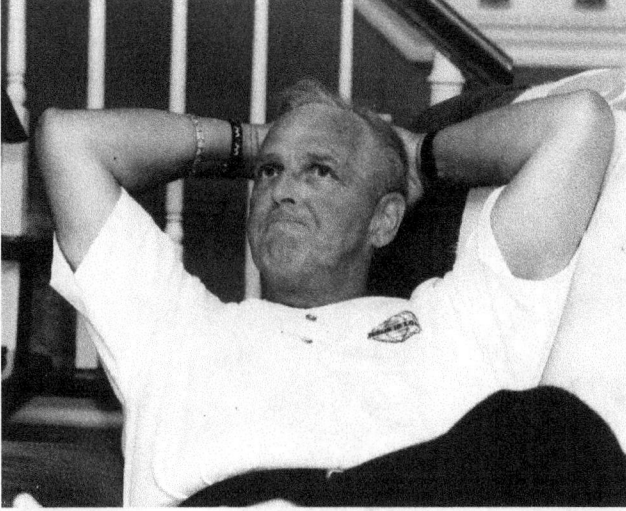

Dad being interviewed by the Anniston Star newspaper. He never took off his "What Would Jesus Do" bracelet. (1999)

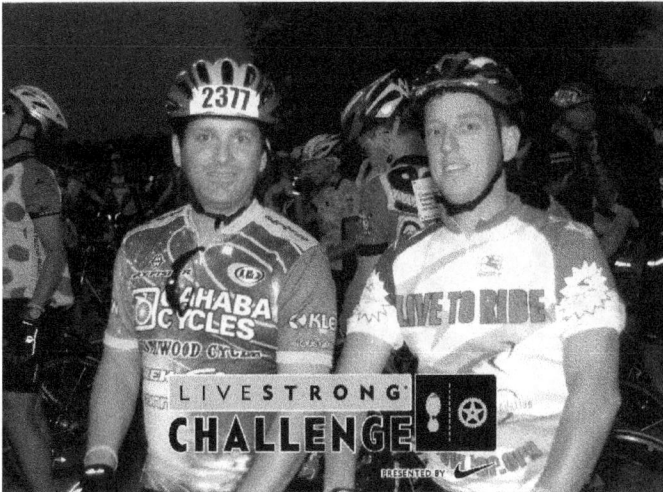

Chatting with a new friend before the 2004 "Ride for the Roses" in Austin, Texas. (October, 2004)

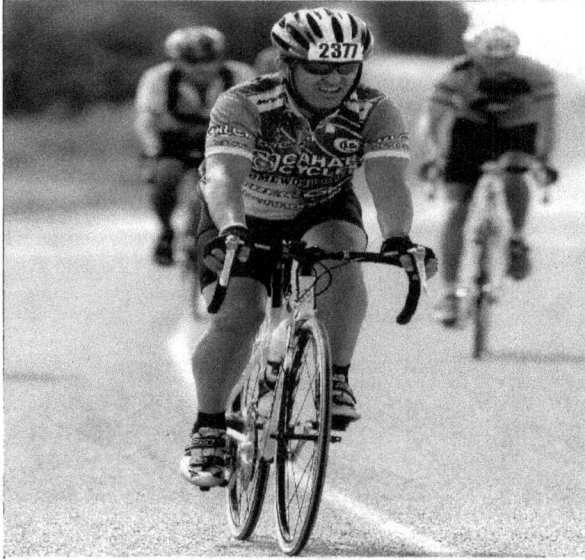

Somewhere between mile one and one hundred in the "Ride for the Roses" in Austin, Texas. (October 2004)

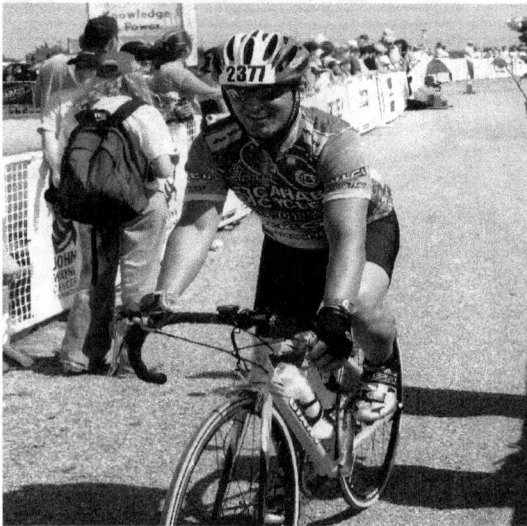

Crossing the finish line at the 2004 "Ride for the Roses" in Austin, Texas. (October 2004)

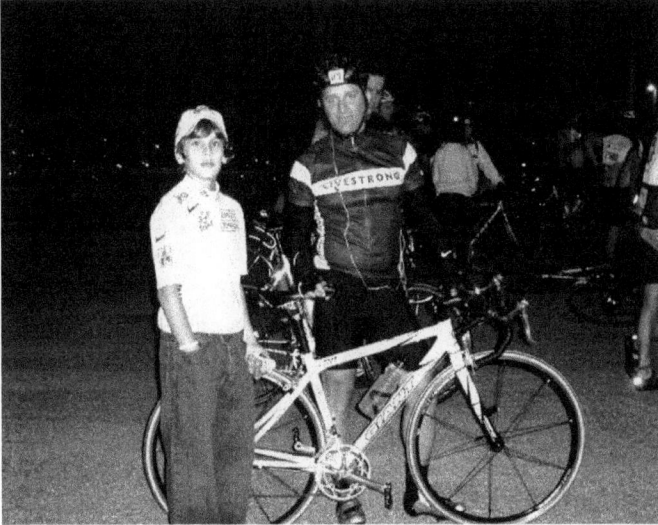

Early morning before the 2005 "Ride for the Roses" in Austin, Texas. Dane was eleven-years-old and was almost as excited as I was to finally be there.

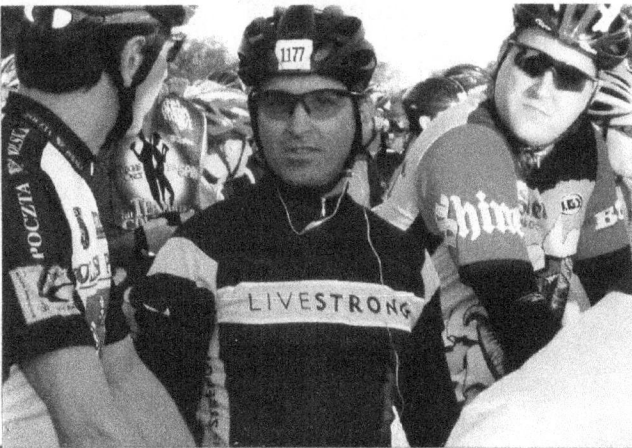

Waiting for the start of the 2005 "Ride for the Roses" in Austin, Texas. I was so excited that Dane was finally here.
(October 2005)

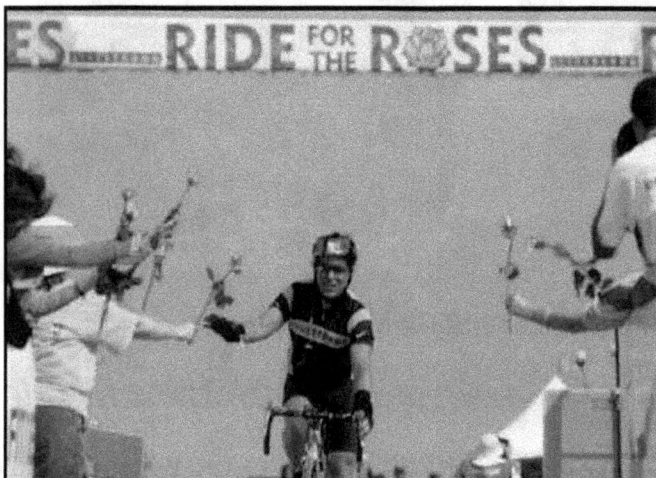

Crossing the finish line at the 2005 "Ride for the Roses". Dane was standing just out of view on the left.

(October 2005)

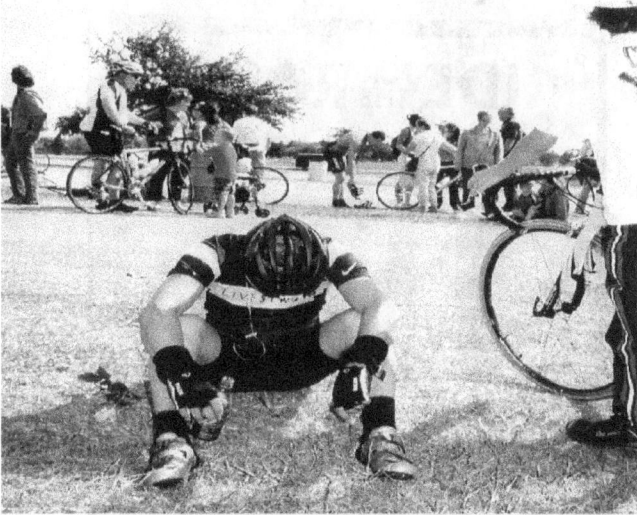

Exhausted and hurting, I'd never been happier. My dream had
come true. Dane, on the right, is holding my bike.
(Austin, Texas - October, 2005)

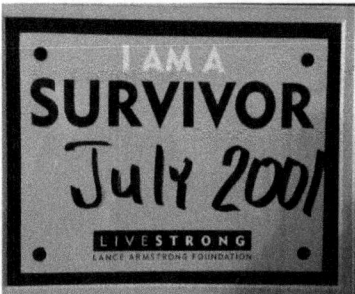

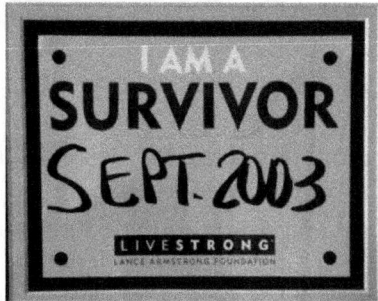

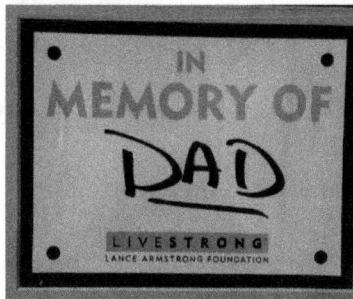

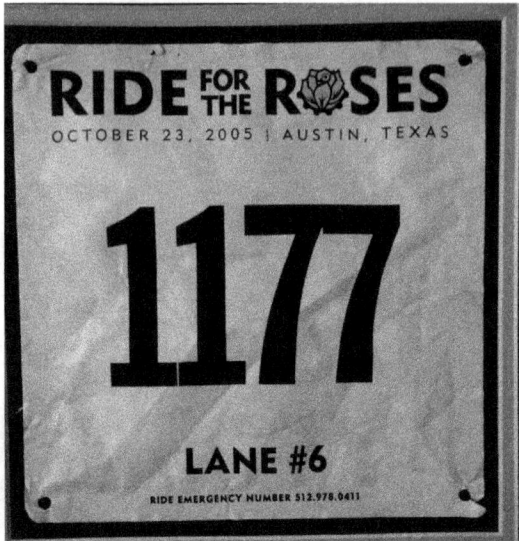

My bib from the 2005 Ride for the Roses and the tags I wore as a survivor and in memory of dad.

On some rides, I would leave the road bike behind and take my mountain bike. My destination would usually be to the end of the paved portion of the Chief Ladiga Trail just east of Piedmont. I would ride the old railroad bed where the rails had been removed and nothing existed but crossties, volcanic scoria, and obsidian rocks. Few people visited that portion of the trail. Just a few miles from the pavement's end toward the Georgia line, I found a special place that provided the only peace I could find during my battle. A small lake that served as an overflow for a nearby watershed sat nestled at the foot of a very steep mountain. With each visit, I would sit down and listen to the sound of nothing but nature and gaze at the beauty of it all. The lake was always perfectly still except for an occasional fish feeding off insects floating on top of the water. The massive mountain behind the lake reflected off the surface like a mirror, making it look even more majestic than it really was. Sitting there in the presence of God's creation, I could reflect on life and death while seeking the true meaning of each. I often wondered if anyone else had ever stopped to notice such a wonderful sight, or would ever know I had visited the place at all. Until then, I'd never appreciated the Appalachian Mountains despite living among them my entire life. The thought of dying among them gave me a whole new appreciation for them.

My cycling continued, and I began showing signs of improvement over the next few weeks and months. The CT scans occurred every four months for the first year. The scans themselves were not bad. Following my scans, I would see Dr. Posey later the same morning to discuss the results. The days leading up to the scans were increasingly stressful. Scan days were simply unbearable. It was pure hell in that examination room waiting, alone, on the results of the CT scans. There wasn't any middle-of-the-road diagnosis when my oncologist came to talk to me about my results. It was either going to be *very* good or *very* bad. But, Doctor Posey always came in, smiled, talked to me about my personal life and my cycling and then proceeded to talk to me about my scans. Each clean scan brought less anxiety for the next one, but they were never easy. I was healthy. I was training. I was eating right, and I felt great.

With almost two years of training as hard as I had ever trained for anything behind me, with so many three and four hour rides behind me, so many hills climbed, and so many roads ridden, I turned into a pretty accomplished cyclist. I had my training and health down to a science, complete with a high antioxidant diet designed to help me push through punishing workouts and help fend off having cancer again. I was the epitome of health. People that never knew about my cancer could not believe I was a survivor.

By October of 2003, my cycling had progressed so much that I was ready for a one-hundred-mile ride in the Ride for the Roses. I had completed several rides of that distance and was finally ready to reach my goal. I had made it…made it to that place I promised myself two years earlier I would be. Life had never been so sweet. I was so giddy the night I registered for the event, I could barely type on my computer from my hands shaking so badly. I made my hotel reservations and could not sleep for thinking about the once-in-a-lifetime event. It was a little over a week away from the Ride for the Roses event, and I decided to cut back the rides and just enjoy what I had accomplished. All I had to left do was have my two-year scans on the Friday before the ride, and then leave for Austin seven days later!

*What are my chances? What do my five-year numbers look like, doc?"*

**LETTERS FROM HEAVEN**

Sitting alone in the waiting room of Kirkland Clinic, I was thinking about the Ride for the Roses and what I needed to pack for my trip. I needed to research more about the actual ride, the hills, how much time it would take me to drive out, and the weather forecasts. I barely heard them call "Tracy Stewart" when it was my turn to see Dr. Posey. I had the familiar weigh-in, blood pressure check, and taking of my temperature as they processed me in and led me to the examination room. I had not been dreading this scan like all the others—up until I was alone in that room. For some reason, I started feeling uneasy…unsure. Where was this coming from? Never before had I actually went down the road of specific thoughts about getting bad news. What if it was bad news? It would be devastating if Dr. Posey walked into the room and told me my cancer had come back and was in my liver—the very thing that killed dad. I started to worry as more and more time elapsed.

When Dr. Posey came into the room, we had our usual chat about cycling and I filled him in about the Ride for the Roses. After a few minutes, he pulled out the chart—as always. As he read the radiologist report, I saw him lean down, as if to indicate, *"Wait. What? What did that say?"* He reached for his pen in his pocket and made a few circles on the report—not like always. A lump came to my throat, and I knew I was in trouble. My heart sank.

"What?" I nervously asked.

"You have a spot in your liver. It is small, and it is the only one that can be seen. You apparently have a reoccurrence." I was stunned. He went on, "I want to schedule a PET scan for you. It will confirm my suspicion of it being cancer."

"What are my chances? What do my five-year numbers look like?" I *knew* the answer before I asked them, but I guess I had to hear it from him anyway.

"About thirty percent. If the PET shows the spot being hot, we will need to talk about options soon."

I knew that those "options" included another surgery, more chemo, and little chance of living a normal life span. I knew that I possibly had a year or two to live. If and when I started going down, it would happen fast—just like dad. I don't remember much after that…not driving…not making a phone call to the office…not making a phone call home. I made it to within a few miles of home, before I noticed I was in Alexandria, Alabama. I didn't have any idea how I got there.

I was about seven miles from home when I pulled over in Lynn Costner's car lot and just broke down into tears. I had been so strong during dad's battle and so strong during my own. How could I fall apart now? I had to pull it together before I got home. I had a nine-year-old at home that had no idea I had been battling cancer for the last two years of his life. After a thirty-minute pity party, I gained my composure and headed home.

I walked into the house and went straight to bed to wallow in my pity quietly. I started feeling guilty about the time I had spent on the bike. I had wasted so much time, not spending it with

Dane. I had to cancel the ride, hang that bike up, and figure out how to make a lifetime of memories in what little time I had left with him. It occurred to me that I should do something that would give Dane a piece of me in the years that followed. I decided to write letters to him and say things that I would say if I were still around. I needed a way to get those to him, but I would have to deal with that later.

The next week, I found myself placed in a room for a PET scan. Apparently, I was going to be so radioactive, I had to wait until medical personnel left the room before I pushed the syringe of solution into the IV. I would have to stay there for two hours before they could come and get me for the scan. It was painless and quick. The results would be known later that day, but I already knew the results. The tests came back conclusive that my cancer was indeed back. I went home and canceled my hotel reservations and the Ride for the Roses. Later that week, I had reservations to visit a chemo infusion center at Kirkland Clinic at UAB.

The following week, I met with Doctor Posey who

prescribed two new drugs—Oxaliplatin and Xeloda. Day one would be an infusion of Oxaliplatin, followed by fourteen days of oral Xeloda, a week off, and then do it all over again. I would stay on this regimen until late November before having an evaluation. During the course of treatment, there would be a couple of CT scans to see if the cancer was reacting to those drugs.

The first infusion of Oxaliplatin was as odd as anything I had ever experienced. The drug felt like how I would imagine liquid nitrogen would feel flowing into your veins. It was freezing cold. During the two-hour infusion, my arm felt like it had been frost bitten. The nurses placed warm packs on my hand and arm, but it had little to no effect. By the time I walked out, my entire arm felt like it had been hit with a hammer and was unusable. Of course, there were side effects to the drug, including extreme sensitivity to cold objects. I could not drink anything below room temperature nor stand in front of a freezer or refrigerator. I was forced to cover my mouth and breathe in my own warm air when outside, and I had to cover my hands with gloves to shield them from the cold. I could not stay outside for long periods of time. The other symptoms involved my jaws locking up, eyes cramping, frequent muscle spasms, and stomach cramps. It was brutal. The first few days after the infusion were difficult, but the sixteen pills a day didn't seem too bad in comparison—except for taking sixteen pills a day.

During the good days, I began to work on my plan for Dane to have something to remember me by. It would be like "Letters from Heaven." I planned to write when I felt like it, and I decided to write a letter for each birthday I would miss, until he was nineteen. I also would write a letter for his first real date, getting his driver's license, his graduation from high school, and for his graduation from college. Of course, I would write one for him to read on his wedding day and one for the birth of his first child. It was very important to me that he never find out where the letters were coming from. I wanted them to show up on his special days. It required finding someone willing to make a lifelong commitment to follow Dane's life and understand how desperately

I needed help. I found the perfect person, but it was important that it would never be revealed to anyone who the letters came from – especially to Dane. Having that resolved instantly put my mind at ease. I was certain Dane would get his letters. My plan was to write them all, then go back and add things I really wanted to say. I didn't know if I would have enough good days to finish them all if I didn't do it that way. At least he would have "something." It would require a lot of writing and time wasn't mine to waste. He was soon going to be ten years old, so I figured I needed to start with his eleventh birthday—just in case. I felt hopeful I would have at least one year left once the surgery was over, but I also knew resecting the liver has a higher mortality rate than my previous surgery. Cutting into an organ that vascular was extremely dangerous. I needed to finish my first letter before my surgery.

*Dane,*

*Today is your eleventh birthday. This is most likely the first letter you have received from me since I left you. There will be many to follow along the way. I guess you can consider them "Letters from Heaven." You will get these from me along your journey in life, at least until you're old enough to understand more about life and why I am not there with you. Don't be angry at God for taking me from you. I spent too much of my life being angry at God. He has a plan for our lives, and this was His plan. Make something great from it!*

*I wanted so badly to see you grow up. I wanted to see you graduate from high school and college, teach you how to drive, watch you play sports, get married, and have your own children. I wanted to be a Paw-Paw to your kids since my dad didn't have much time to be yours. If it were up to me, I would have been there for all those things! I also want you to know how hard I tried to beat the cancer. I never stopped fighting it. You were the reason— the only reason really—that I kept pushing myself in my battle.*

*Just because I am not there doesn't mean I am not with you each and every day. I may not be physically there to witness those things in your life, but I can still share them with you. Love still lives in our hearts after someone dies and that is for a reason. I cannot imagine God would have you here loving me, without it working both ways. I am certain I will be able to share in your life and help watch over you as you grow up.*

*Also, I can sense Paw-Paw's presence around me so often—usually when I am alone. So, even when you can't see me or hear me, I hope you sit still long enough to feel my presence around you. Don't be sad for me, because I am okay. Besides, life it way too short to be sad, and I want you to be happy every moment of your life. Always remember to smile and laugh and live life one day at a time. Make a point every day to seek happiness. It is the key to living a good life. Know too that I am very proud of you and know you will make something great of yourself! Whatever you decide to do—in anything—give it your best shot.*

*Life goes by really quickly and we will see each other again. You have a full life to live, so live it to the fullest and know that I will be waiting on you where there won't be any more good-byes.*

*Always know that I love you with all my heart!*

*—Dad*

I had so much more to say, but I knew there would be many letters to write if I made it through the surgery.

Once it was confirmed my cancer was reacting to the new drugs, my next surgery was scheduled for December 17. My next doctor's visit was the following week, and I was assigned my third UAB physician, a surgical oncologist named Dr. Martin Heslin. He was an Ivy League guy and one of the best at what he did. In fact, I had read about some of the clinical trials he had participated in and knew the name already.

The meeting with Doctor Heslin was an interesting one. He was about my age and rather small in stature. As soon as I met him, my first words were, "I have to know something, doc. How did you go from being a college wrestler at Cornell to a surgeon at UAB?"

It was my attempt to make this "personal" with him too. It seemed to work with my other two oncologists. If a surgeon was going to be cutting on me, I wanted to know all about this person, and I wanted him to know all about me.

He grinned and said, "So you've been doing your homework. I wanted to go to an Ivy League school, and being a college wrestler was the only way I was going to get in."

I thought how he didn't seem like a wrestler. But he had an aura of confidence about him that I rarely have experienced with any other person in my life. It was borderline cocky, but not. It was certainly a trait that I was looking for, because I needed him to be assured of what he was doing. His demeanor seemed to put me at ease, and I knew I was in great hands.

He began. "What you have is a single, small lesion in your liver. What have you been told or read about your prognosis?"

"Thirty percent." I felt confident in saying it. I had read that on many Web sites and even had been told that by Dr. Posey.

Dr. Heslin responded. "I am going to say it is probably a little higher than that. You have a single lesion and it is smaller than five centimeters, which is a plus one. You don't have any other lesions, which is a plus one. Your Carcinoembryonic Antigen test, which measures protein in your blood and serves as a tumor marker, shows your levels are not elevated. That is a plus one. Your recurrence happened two years later, which is a plus one. The cancer is confined to your liver, which is a plus one. So, you have five plus ones. I looked at your scans, and they are showing your cancer is highly sensitive to the drugs we have prescribed, but I am taking you off them now because I am afraid we won't be able to find it when we resection your liver. I am going to take this lesion out and be done with it." He was so confident. That was the most unbelievable thing he could have said to me. It was so hard to believe. I began to question it, but I wanted to believe it.

*God, I don't know what you want from me, but I can't stand it any longer. I have not slept in seven nights, and I have not eaten in six days. I am in constant pain, and I can't take it anymore."*

## THE LEDGE AND THE LAST PROMISE

The seventeenth of December came much sooner than I had imagined. The pre-surgery chemo had ended and Dr. Heslin made the appointment for the surgery.

On the morning of the surgery, Dr. Heslin came by to check on me in the prep room. I was later moved into a holding area with others and connected to vital sign monitors. TVs were arranged for us to watch, but I didn't care much for watching. I knew what waited for me on the backside of the surgery and it was ugly. It would be days and nights filled with more pain, more scars, and more staples. At least the first time, I didn't know what to expect. Now, I knew exactly what to expect.

I was later wheeled into the operating room and was amazed at what I was seeing. It looked like something from inside a UFO in a sci-fi movie. I had been asleep before entering the operating room on my previous surgery. There was so much equipment. I could not believe it.

One of the surgeons came in and asked if I would be okay if they strapped my arms out crucifix style.

I replied, "I think this will be the *least* of what you all are about to do to me."

He laughed. "You are probably correct."

Doctor Heslin came in shortly afterward, covered with scrubs, a mask, and goggles to match. "Let's do this."

With that, the backward counting started. "One hundred...ninety-nine...ninety..." and that was it.

The next thing I heard was, "Wake up sleepy head. Are you going to wake up for me? Sweetie, are you going to talk to me? Open those eyes for me."

It was an ICU nurse talking to me. I was confused, but I knew I was in pain and that it would be getting worse. I don't know how long I was in recovery, but I was eventually taken to a room. I was finally able to wake up enough to look at my abdomen for the large incision. Sure enough, it was there, only longer and running at a forty-five-degree angle from the scar of my previous surgery. The pain this time around wasn't a piece of cake, but this time the UAB doctors had inserted a device that contained a small vial of medicine along the incision area to assist with pain management. It did nothing to mask the devastation of looking at another long incision held together by thirty-eight staples.

The day following my surgery, Dr. Heslin came to see me and explained they had to take out the complete right lobe of my liver.

"We couldn't find the tumor when we got in there. The drugs had done a number on your tumor. We couldn't take the chance of doing a resection not knowing where it was, so we took half your liver. We finally found the spot once we had that part of your liver out, but we had a hard time seeing it. We know your cancer is very sensitive to these drugs, so you will go back on them for a while after the first of the year."

Five days later, on December 23, 2003, the nurses came in that morning to inform me that I was being discharged. I honestly didn't feel my body was ready, but I sure wanted to go home in the worst way. I was instructed to get dressed, and the nurse removed my morphine pump. I dressed and sat in a chair thinking it would be soon. I waited and waited but no doctor made rounds to sign my release papers. The hours ticked by like molasses. At 3 p.m. I was hurting. They had written me a prescription for pain, but I couldn't get released from the hospital to get it filled. I was informed they could not give me any medications on the day I got dismissed, so I just sat there and dealt with the pain. My nurse kept coming back to the room to check on me, and each time she got angrier that I was forced to sit there in pain with no means to do anything about it. She was angry the doctors had forced me off the IV-fed morphine and given me no alternate means of medicating for so long. A doctor finally made rounds at 4 p.m., but I was in such pain by that time that I literally threw up trying to get up to walk. I was wheeled to the car and sent on my way.

The ride from Birmingham, Alabama, to home took significantly longer due to an eight mile out of the way stop at Jim 'N Nick's BBQ for dinner. It wasn't of my choosing. I was hurting too much to eat and just wanted to get home. This trip was over two hours long and the constant "bump-de-bump-de-bump" of the car bouncing across the expansion joints on the interstate was very painful. By the time I got home, I felt as though I would pass out from the weakness and pain. I climbed into bed hoping for some relief. It was the day before Christmas Eve, and I had not even told my mom or that side of the family that I'd had a recurrence— or surgery for that matter. I planned on telling them when we visited on Christmas Day and after the surgery was a success. There was no sense in ruining the holidays for them too. In hindsight, this was probably a selfish choice on my part. I should have told my mother at least.

It turned out that I wasn't going to make it for the annual Christmas visit. I was in too much pain, cut half in two, depressed, and unable to eat or sleep.

UAB had scheduled my chemo to resume in early January, and I had some serious healing to do before that started again. I can't explain how badly I didn't want to go back on chemo, but at least I was home.

The comfort of home, though, wasn't all that comforting. The pain pills were useless. I was already in pain before I even got home, and once I got behind on pain medication, there was no catching up.

Five days after returning home, I was still bedridden. I had not slept a single second because of the amount of pain I was in, nor had I eaten because of the swelling and bloating I was experiencing. Apparently my digestive system wasn't waking up, or it had fallen back asleep after my surgery. The last solid food I had eaten was given to me the day before I left the hospital and it never digested. It went to my stomach and just sat there. Some bloating or swelling after abdominal surgery can be expected, but my belly was protruding like a woman's in her third trimester. The pain was never ceasing and was so intense my ears were literally ringing, and the lack of food only made me weaker. I was in a bad situation—too exhausted to get out of bed and too bloated to eat for energy. Pain medication wasn't an option because it slows the digestive track and mine was stopped completely.

I can't explain what it is like to experience a twenty-four hour torture episode that went on day-after-day-after-day, but with no sleep. I became suicidal.

By the seventh day, and without one second of relief, I simply couldn't go on living with the constant pain and wanted to die. Late into the evening, I laid in bed contemplating my options on how to relieve myself of the pain. I had a 9mm Ruger pistol in the bedroom closet and thought about ending it that way. But, there was a nine-year-old little boy sleeping in another room down the hall. A tragic event like that would have scarred him for life. It would always be the house his father ended his life in and that would not have been fair to him. I had the pain pills left over from the surgery and considered taking those, but I only had eight left— certainly not enough to do the job. I had no options to ease the unrelenting pain. By 2 a.m. that morning, I finally slid out of bed and onto the floor. I'm not sure what I was trying to accomplish. I just needed help and couldn't lie there any longer. Unable to help myself and with no one to turn to, it was time I had the long-awaited reckoning with God. It was just me and Him. I eventually crawled to my knees and held the edge of the bed.

*"God, I don't know what you want from me, but I can't stand this any longer. Please take me out of this world. I would rather die if this is the life I have to live. Just take me now. I am in constant pain. I tried to beat this by myself but I couldn't. I wanted to live long enough to see Dane grow up. I wanted to see him get married and get to know his kids. I wanted to see him graduate from high school. I wanted to live long enough that he would be able to remember me. Do with me what you will, but if you don't help me tonight, I am ending this somehow. Please, God, help me...stop the pain... just let me sleep."*

I was on the border of insanity and teetering on the ledge between this life and the next. Something had to give. It seemed odd that I was asking for God's help. I had not spoken to Him since dad passed away four years earlier. I had been too angry and too stubborn to give in.

I pulled myself back into bed and immediately found the pain subsiding—just like that. I went to sleep within a few minutes and woke up five hours later feeling amazingly energetic. I couldn't believe how much had changed within a few hours. The pain was still there, but it had subsided to "manageable." I was experiencing God's Grace. Maybe that was what God wanted all along—for me to just leave it with Him and have faith that He would take care of everything…the pain…the worry…the cancer. My approach to my battle and how I would live my life after that night would never be the same. God brought me to a place where He was the only answer. Complete faith in God was the gift from having cancer.

The next morning, I decided I would start walking to see if I could reduce some of the bloating and get my digestive track going again. Our mailbox was two-tenths of a mile from the front steps. A round trip there and back was almost a half-mile walk. I thought, *If I am not back in twenty minutes, somebody better come looking for me,* and I walked out the door. It took me nearly that long to make the short trek. I was so weak. But the more I walked, the less pain I had. I literally crawled up the front steps and into the house before collapsing on the sofa. I slept for almost five hours, and repeated the walk that afternoon. The day before, I could not have walked the length of the house, much less made that walk to the mailbox. The difference was I wasn't walking alone—not anymore. The poem "Footprints in the Sand" is all about God carrying us when we can't make it ourselves, but you have to allow Him to. He wanted to carry me all along. That morning on my knees, I finally allowed him to pick me up into his arms. I let Him carry me. Never again would I worry about my fate or my cancer.

I was finally able to get some strength just in time to be pounded again with chemo on January 4. I stayed on chemo until the first week of March of 2004.

April arrived and with it some warmer weather. With the side effects of chemo waning, I started increasing my time outdoors. I wanted to absorb life and spend as much time with Dane as I possibly could. I didn't want to return to work or do anything that would take me away from him. If God did allow me to live until he graduated from high school, I needed to get busy making memories.

I had decided the training, the bike, and Austin was only a dream and no longer a good one. I wasn't going to get back on. I was angry at myself and full of regret for spending all of that time on the bike after my first diagnosis. How selfish could I have been? All this time I had focused on being on that bike, training to be able to ride one-hundred miles with Lance Armstrong, and I missed what was most important of all—time with Dane.

One April afternoon, Dane and I were cleaning out the garage. We were being silly and having some quality father-son time. I was embracing the time with him when Dane walked over to my Giant TCR bike hanging on the wall. I noticed him standing there staring at it. He turned toward me and looked at me with his big, brown eyes.

"Are you gonna start riding your bike again?"

I had an easy answer. "No. I don't think I will."

Dane looked surprised and confused. "I thought you were going to ride with Lance Armstrong in Austin. Are you never gonna ride ever again?"

I just stood there speechless, sensing that he was really asking much more. I realized Dane had watched me fight for so long, even if he didn't know what I was fighting or that my life was in jeopardy. He was now watching me quit. It would probably be how he remembered me later in his life.

"Dane, do you know what is wrong with me?" I asked. I suspected he did.

"You have cancer like Paw-Paw." I could sense he was looking for some reassurance and confidence in my voice—just like I was that day I walked into dad's hospital room seven years earlier.

At first, I didn't know how to handle the conversation so I just let it flow in hopes of picking his brain as to what he was thinking. "How long have you known?"

"I don't know. A long time." His eyes shifted away. I knew he was worried that his dad's fate would be the same as my own dad's had been.

I looked over at the bike. Dust had accumulated on the rims and seat. The tires were completely flat. Suddenly, as if God Himself had planted an idea and the words that followed, I said, "Dane, if I get you a road bike like mine, would you ride with me?" It was a way that I could fight the disease, for him to share in my battle, *and* still spend quality time with him. It was the perfect solution.

He turned back toward me and his eyes lit up. "Yeah, I would love that. Will you really buy me one?" A big grin came across his face.

My heart was content as I offered, "Yeah, I will. When I get my bike fixed up, we'll go get you one."

I was happy. I knew I had to start the fight again, even if I started from less than nothing. I said I was going to Austin, and I needed to go. It may be the most memorable thing Dane would ever see me do, and I may have only *one* shot at it.

"I *promise* you, Dane, I am getting back on that bike and I *will* go to Austin. And you will see me cross that finish line." As it parted my lips, I wondered if it was a promise I could keep.

*I knew from that moment on it would be me and Dane in this fight. He hadn't given up on me, and I hadn't given up on me either.*

## AUSTIN

Over the next few months I trained as much as my health would allow. I would ride with Dane each afternoon that he wanted to ride, just to get a few miles in. It was like starting over—maybe worse. Our afternoon rides would last as long as the sun allowed. Saturday and Sunday mornings were filled with three or four hour rides alone, usually beginning at 6:30 a.m. I would get some serious training in while Dane was still asleep. If he wanted to go when I got back, we'd head back out for a ride together later in the day. Weather was never a factor in my training. If the sun was shining, I was riding; if it was raining, I was riding. I wasn't sure I would make it to Austin—if I made it at all—but I certainly trained like it. The October 2004 Ride for the Roses would be my best chance to do it. I *had* to make it somehow, someway.

My legs remembered what it took to be a rider that could push a bike one-hundred miles. It was never easy cranking the pedals roughly 30,000 times, but my progress came at a much faster pace than before.

By September, it was obvious all the training had paid off. It had been less than a year since I canceled the 2003 ride, but it seemed so much longer. The surgery, chemo, and training had prevented me from being on the bike during four of those months. It was the most challenging time in my life, but once again I was ready to head out to Austin.

I made my reservations for the Austin ride in late September. I couldn't wait to share the news to Dane that I was really going to make it there this time. My excitement was short lived when I was informed I would be making the trip alone. My wife opted out of going—claiming Dane would have to miss two days of school. I knew that wasn't the reason, but it was the excuse she used. I could not fathom how she could stand in the way of something so monumentally important to me or to Dane. It was a sign of things to come, and I knew from that moment on it would only be me and Dane in my fight. He hadn't given up on me, and I hadn't given up on me either.

Without his mother there to watch him while I complete the ride, Dane would not be able to go with me. I couldn't leave him for five or six hours alone, hoping he would be there at the finish line when I returned. He had been the driving force behind every turn of the crank I'd made and every drop of sweat I'd poured out. He was in every heartbeat that pumped oxygen to my muscles when I had labored for air. It was his face I saw on my long rides that left me depleted of every ounce of energy I had. I endured every drop of chemotherapy that was infused into my veins because of that kid, and I wanted more than anything in this world for him to be there with me. But that was taken from him—and from me. Not going wasn't an option. I could not miss the only opportunity to complete a journey I might never have the chance to pursue again. Even going without him, Dane would know I set out to accomplish something that 99 percent of people on earth couldn't do. He would know I wasn't afraid to dream big, work hard, and finish something I set out to do. He could take that with him throughout his life.

On October 15, I packed my bags, loaded up my bike, and headed out for Austin, Texas, alone. Every mile I drove of that 900 miles and every minute of that thirteen-hour trip, were heartbreaking as Dane filled my thoughts. I drove the entire trip in one day.

Arriving in Austin, I couldn't believe how many bikes I saw on the road and on bike racks. It was insane. Checking into the hotel, I saw rider after rider walking their bikes to their rooms. Electricity filled the air as I went to check into my hotel. That evening in the lobby I struck up a conversation with two cyclists from California. Jim worked for a tech company, and David worked in marketing. It was their first trip to the Ride for the Roses too. They were stereotypical Californians - long blonde hair, wayfarer sunglasses, and repeatedly referred to me as "dude". I was a typical Alabamian with my deep southern accent, a passion for college football, and was little smarter than I appeared to be. We had nothing in common except the passion for cycling, but that was enough, and we hit it off immediately. When they discovered I was a cancer survivor and had made the trip alone, they invited me to go to dinner with them. We shared some interesting cycling stories and promised to meet up somewhere at the event and ride together.

The next day, cyclists were instructed to pick up their ride packages at the conference, which included a map of the ride, my bib, some coupons, and some reading material about cancer. My hands shook as I gazed at my bib number for the first time. I met Lance's mom, Linda, at the event. It was so cool finally meeting her after reading so much about her in Lance's book. I noticed how almost every single person I saw there had people supporting them, encouraging them, and sharing in their journey. I would have loved having Dane there to experience what I was about to do. It would have been easy to allow my anger of him not being there steal my moment and my joy, but this was too important. I'd come way too far, worked way too long, and prayed often to be where I was.

That night I attended an open-forum interview that Ann Curry was doing with Lance. I decided to walk to the event since it was only about a mile away from my hotel. On my way back, I stopped at the Congress Avenue Bridge and took in the world's largest urban bat colony. I sat on a bench nearby and talked with Dad for a while. I felt his presence so strongly that night. Maybe it was being in Texas again, but he felt nearer and closer to me. I needed his guidance and his wisdom so badly. It was clear that my life would be changing with or without cancer. I went back to the hotel with a heavy heart.

On October 17, 2004, I woke up early and got my cycling gear ready. I loaded my energy drinks on the bike and packed energy bars and GU packs in my jersey pockets. I sat quietly for the longest time in the solitude of that hotel room. I'd never felt more alone in this world. I pinned two signs on the back of my jersey. One read "In memory of Dad" and the other "I am a

Survivor—September 2003." On my left calf, a henna tattoo read "Courage" and on the right calf, "Strength." My left wrist donned "Dane," and my right wrist had the word "Dad," both written with a black Sharpie. I loaded the bike and made my way to the Travis County Convention Center where I took my place among 6,500 cyclists. I'd never seen anything like the sea of bright, colored, cycling jerseys stretching across the distance. The chutes were broken into divisions by the various distances cyclists were attempting. I quickly found the 100-mile chute and noticed it was significantly smaller than the others. Maybe I was biting off more than I could chew. I panned the riders looking for my newfound friends from California but saw neither.

I stood there taking it all in when I heard, "Hey, Bama! Where are you from?"

I was confused for a second as a man approached me.

"I saw your jersey and immediately noticed it was a Cahaba Cycles Jersey. Are you from Birmingham?"

I explained that I was from Jacksonville, was there as a cancer survivor, and was alone. He wasn't even riding the event, but had come to cheer on a loved one. We chatted for a while and he went back to his family. It was nice knowing at least one other person from Alabama was there, but it gave me a longing for home.

As starting time neared, Lance Armstrong, Sheryl Crow, and Will Ferrell appeared at the start line to welcome the cyclists. Families and friends were all smiles, taking pictures of their cyclists who were riding in memory of (or in honor of) someone they loved. I'm sure many were also survivors like me, but there would be no photos of me unless the professional photographers, hired by the event coordinators, happened to snap a few of me along the way.

The ride began at the sound of a gun. The one-hundred-milers were the last chute to leave the starting line. When we reached US Highway 290, there were cyclists riding four and five wide, spanning miles ahead of me. The pace was quicker than I was accustomed to and surprisingly easy to maintain. I'd trained almost three years either riding alone and without the assistance of drafting, or allowing Dane to draft behind me. Considering there was a significant headwind, it was a good thing there was a draft to be in. It was a little unnerving being inches from another cyclist's back wheel, who I didn't even know, hoping he wouldn't suddenly hit his breaks. The road wound through Austin's Hill Country. Occasionally a rest stop would appear with cyclists standing around talking and taking in nourishment. I passed the first one, then the second without stopping. I was there to finish something and didn't want to lose the draft of the group I was riding in. As the ride continued, I saw signs detouring for the various distances…10 miles…25 miles…40 miles…I just kept turning the cranks. I glanced down at my cyclometer and noticed I'd been riding an hour and thirty minutes. I switched the cyclometer to "average mph" and noticed it was just over twenty-six miles per hour, which was much faster than my training rides.

As I neared the seventy-mile detour, I noticed the number of riders had diminished to a handful. I was riding in a group of about fourteen cyclists. Most of them were with Trek Travel. About half the riders took the seventy-mile detour. The half I went with dropped me from their draft shortly after the detour. I started taking in my GU packs and energy bars for nourishment, wishing I had made at least one of the rest stops. Without drafting partners, the Texas winds were taking what little power I had left in my legs. My legs began to cramp so badly I could hardly spin the pedals. I knew if I stopped, that would be it. If I bonked, there would be nobody there to push me through it. Occasionally I would pass a cyclist or one would pass me. We would draft together for a while, and then continue at our respective paces. Somewhere in that desolate Texas prairie, I began to settle into riding alone. It had been the way I trained and was familiar to me. I felt a comforting spirit around me as my cramping legs began to feel refreshed and my labored breathing became at ease. It was just the four of us—God, me, Dane, and dad.

A few miles farther into my ride, a town appeared. The streets were empty and all of the stores were closed. It looked like a ghost town. Not a single person was stirring, but there was music playing loudly. As I entered the center of that small Texas town, I could make out the song. It was the Pointer Sisters' "I'm So Excited." I turned a corner at the end of town and there was a huge gazebo with people scurrying about everywhere. A few cyclists had stopped before me to rest and take on food and drink. It looked like the entire town had come out to welcome the weary cyclists that took on the one-hundred-mile ride. Grown men danced around in pink outfits with high heels and yellow bolos around their necks. Occasionally, they would venture into the crowd as they lip synched the words and flirted with the cyclists. I pulled over, joined the festivities, and rested my aching legs. I sat and watched these crazy fellows and laughed at their antics as I sucked on oranges and ate fig bars. It was so refreshing to see how these people supported cancer survivors and their loved ones. They went all out for the event. As much as I wanted to stay and visit, the road called my name and it was time to finish what I came to do. I hopped back on the bike for the last ten to fifteen miles of my journey.

With refreshed legs, I sped away as the music faded in the distance. In what seemed like only minutes, I glanced down one last time to my cyclometer to check the mileage—101.6 miles. I raised my eyes from the road to see a welcome site a short distance away. The top of the Travis County Convention Center stood just beyond a tree line. Putting my head back down and ducking into an aerodynamic position, I pushed the pedals with what strength I had left in me. The Texas heat and thirty-mile-an-hour winds had beaten me up all day, and I wanted to finish strong. As I entered the fair grounds and made my last turn, I looked up to see hundreds of people cheering me on. Ladies stood lining each side of the entrance with yellow shirts and holding yellow roses for the riders. I had been told there would be a surprise at the end of the ride, but I had not expected that at all. Tears rolled down my cheeks as I made my last push toward the finish line. At 1:35 p.m. on October

17, 2004, I took my yellow rose, pounded my chest with my fist, and pointed to the heavens, *"For you dad..."*

Many years of fight, struggle, and pain lay along my journey to get to that place and time. My fight had come full circle. I did it. But it was bittersweet. There should have been someone waiting and watching for me to complete that journey...someone that wanted to be there and someone that I wanted to be there more than anything in this world. I crossed the finish line unaccompanied, but I was more certain than ever that I was not in the fight alone anymore. Dane was in it with me and so was God. I walked my bike over to a large field, laid it down, and used the saddle for a pillow. I looked around at all the people celebrating with family and friends. They were laughing and having a festive time surrounded by those they loved. I smiled, shut my eyes, and reflected on the magnitude of it all. I thought, *I need to forget about writing those "Letters from Heaven." I'm going to be okay. I will just tell him all those things myself.*

My thoughts turned to dad and all the things he taught me. I swung at a bad pitch and hit a home run. I felt I had beaten my cancer, but only because he didn't. His dying of cancer was the reason I went for a checkup. It saved my life. Every single fight we made together in his battle, every website I visited, every stone I overturned, everything thing I had researched, was God's way of preparing me for my own battle.

*I dismounted from the bike as Dane came over to hug me. He had no idea how long I'd waited for that to happen.*

## THE JOURNEY CONTINUES

There was only one small thing left undone in my journey. I still needed to fulfill a promise I had made to a brown-eyed, little boy in our garage one April morning.

I continued to train the next year, and I would ride with Dane as often as time would allow. Together, we rode thousands of miles in the scorching hot sun, gusty winds, pouring rains, and bitter cold. He stayed with me pedal-for-pedal on most of my rides, often forcing me to keep up, as he became an accomplished rider himself. During our rides, he was able to share in the experience of that peace and tranquility I felt riding through the Appalachian Mountains on the Chief Ladiga Trail. The pavement of the trail just east of Piedmont was completed, so we would often ride to Georgia on our road bikes. We would always stop at that special place with the lake, and I would tell him stories about my previous visits and why that place was so special to me. I wanted this to be a place Dane could come and hopefully feel my presence if I lost my battle with cancer.

On October 23, 2005, I was back in Austin once more to ride the one-hundred-mile event, only this time Dane was with me. Our riding together created a bond that was even stronger than we had before and allowed him to feel like he was more a part of my journey. He still wasn't ready for one-hundred miles in the hills of Austin, Texas, so he would sit this ride out. But he was there to experience what a person can accomplish with perseverance and determination and would be there waiting at the finish line when I crossed it. Most importantly, it would be something he would always remember. He would know that like me, he was a part of his dad's battle with cancer.

The Ride for the Roses that afternoon was much more difficult than the previous year. Significant wind gusts had riders off their bikes and lying on the sides of the roads exhausted and cramping. Rider after rider opted out of the longer rides, leaving very few drafting partners in the last stages. It didn't help that I was also riding with cracked ribs—thanks to a mountain bike crash two weeks before the event. Every deep breath I took sent sharp pains through my left ribcage, so I focused on shallow, quick breaths to allow enough oxygen to fuel my ride.

As the miles clicked by, I took notice of how many of the riders were actually cancer survivors. Most of these people were not veteran cyclists either, and to see them methodically cranking those pedals mile-after-mile-after-mile is awe-inspiring – even to a fellow survivor. Cancer survivors know more about pain and determination than any cyclists I've ever met. Even though the Texas winds and hill country were no pieces of cake, they paled in comparison to what those survivors had pushed through while battling their diseases. At the mark for the turn to the seventy-mile ride, I wanted desperately to follow the riders in front of me as they all made that turn. But I had come too far to not push another thirty miles. I was the only rider in sight that stayed on the one-hundred-mile course. It would just be me for a while—just like the last Ride for the Roses. Eventually, I caught up with another rider as we took turns drafting and shielding the wind gusts off of each other. We were both so exhausted; we never spoke a word to each other. It was just a mutual understanding that we needed each other to get to the end. Around mile ninety, we were caught up by a group of about ten riders and they sucked us into their draft. I knew if I could just stay in the draft I'd be okay, but all the miles I had pushed through the winds alone had left my legs cramping and powerless. I had only ridden with the group for a couple of miles when we came to a railroad track that crossed the road at a bit of an angle. I had shifted out of the drafting line to fall back into the pack about the time we crossed the track. It was just enough of an angle difference for the slick iron rail to send my front tire sliding down the tracks and me sliding down the asphalt. The group stopped to check on me, but I was okay. I reinjured my ribs, suffered some road rash, and a bruised ego, but otherwise, I was lucky to walk away mostly unharmed. I told the group to go ahead without me, and I knew my draft would be gone for the last seven or eight miles of the ride. I was already aching all over just from being on the bike that long. While checking out my bike and before mounting the saddle again, my phone rang. It was Dane.

"Dad, where are you? I thought you would be here by now."

Doing my best impression of a rider that wasn't hurting or struggling to finish, I explained, "I'll be there shortly. I had an accident, but I'm okay and about to get back on the bike."

"How much longer?" Dane had about as much patience as I did, which is none.

Unsure, I replied with a safe estimate. "Maybe thirty minutes. Just be at the start finish line. It won't be any longer than that."

The rest of the ride was more painful than any I had ever spent on a bike or in training. The last mile included that long climb which requires some serious lung capacity and the ability to ride through cramping. There were more riders on the side of the road or pushing than in the saddle turning pedals. I tried to focus on Dane standing there at the finish line, waiting to see me cross. I had waited four long years for that to happen and it was the driving force in my return to Austin. It was enough to get me through.

Soon, the familiar site of the Travis County fairgrounds came into view. I had nothing left in me to finish strong or for any sprint at the end like I had the previous year. I took my rose and made the last turn into the fairgrounds. As I coasted toward the finish line, I spotted Dane and his white baseball cap, standing there waiting for me. It was a vision I'd dreamed about for so long. It just took two trips to Austin, two surgeries, three chemotherapy drugs, fourteen months of treatments, twenty-eight rounds of radiation, and thousands of miles of training to see it.

I dismounted from the bike as Dane came over to hug me. He had no idea how long I'd waited for that to happen. He took my bike and walked it toward the truck as we talked about the ride, the wreck, and what he'd done while he waited on me. For the first time since July 11, 2001, I felt complete and perfectly content.

# FINAL THOUGHTS

Rarely are we given second chances in life. It is even rarer to be given a third. But when we are, we live stronger and love deeper than we ever thought possible. I have found that everything in life is green again, and every experience I encounter is like the first time. Each day I feel like a child waking up on Christmas morning who finds a brand new bike under the tree. Living out my days with the faith that God is in control is like letting go of the handlebars and riding with no hands. It is scary at first, but the freedom and excitement in doing so is unexplainable.

The years have passed much too quickly, and Dane has grown into a young man. He is now a freshman in college at Jacksonville State University majoring in Business Administration. I've lived those years one day at a time and savored moments in each and every one. I will always do so too. I seek happiness in each and every day, and I find it.

Before I was diagnosed with cancer, I was walking through life as if my only objective was to just get to the end of it. I believed life was meant to be comfortable, and I often surrounded myself with people and things that were considered safe and simple. A fulfilled life doesn't work that way at all, but it is how most of us live our lives. A void existed in my life because very few of my life experiences were of my own seeking or doing. I just happened to be there when they occurred. Recognizing the opportunities to experience life is one thing; however, seeking out opportunities to experience what life has to offer is something totally different. When I view life through retrospective glasses, I realize that there was a script for life that I believed I was expected to follow. It was to go to school, then to college, start a career, get married, have kids, have grandkids, retire, and die. I treated each phase of my life as if I was waiting for the next one to begin. When the next phase came, I expected it to be better because God owed that to me. I did nothing significant to add to the gift of life in any stage I was currently in.

God's blessed me with a gift of knowing how to live life to the fullest. In my most desperate time, God carried me. It was His footprints in the sand. He was with me during my entire battle, waiting for me to reach out to Him. I never had a complete understanding of the true meaning of faith until cancer called. I'm far from perfect, but my faith in God is so strong that I know His will in my life determines when my time will come. God left me here longer than I asked of Him, and I've been blessed beyond measure by Him doing so. I've had more time to make life-long memories with my son, Dane.

I was also blessed by starting my life over with a remarkable woman. My wife, Brigett, is the most amazing woman I've ever known. Like me, she has an incredible passion in all that she does and completely understands what is important in life. She possesses incredible strength and loves me despite my many flaws. She is my rock when I'm on shaky ground and is in it for the long haul. She doesn't give up on me or opt out when trouble finds us. I've heard many survivors question why God left them here among the living, but it isn't something I will ever question. I know why He left me here. I know why I didn't die from my disease….

… It was not on His agenda either.

www.ingramcontent.com/pod-product-compliance
Lightning Source LLC
Chambersburg PA
CBHW050121280326
41933CB00010B/1198